CONQUER TYPE 2 DIABETES WITH A KETOGENIC DIET

A Practical Guide for Reducing Your HBA1c and Avoiding Diabetic Complications

ELLEN DAVIS ◆ KEITH RUNYAN

Gutsy Badger Publishing
Cheyenne, Wyoming

Ellen Davis, MS
Gutsy Badger Publishing
Cheyenne, Wyoming
Email: ask.ellen.davis@gmail.com
Website: www.ketogenic-diet-resource.com

All of the information provided in and throughout this book (hereafter known as Publication) and offered at http://www.ketogenic-diet-resource.com is intended solely for general information and should NOT be relied upon for any particular diagnosis, treatment, or care. This is not a substitute for medical advice or treatment. This Publication and the website are only for general informational purposes. It is strongly encouraged that individuals and their families consult with qualified medical professionals for treatment and related advice on individual cases before beginning any diet. The full legal disclaimer is located in appendix E.

Conquer Type 2 Diabetes with a Ketogenic Diet / Ellen Davis and Keith Runyan

ISBN 978-1-943721-06-1   Paperback
ISBN 978-1-943721-08-5   Ebook

To everyone struggling with the harsh reality of a diabetes diagnosis and, especially, to my mother, who died of diabetic complications and liver cancer at the young age of sixty-three. I wish with all my heart that I had known then what I know now.

Ellen Davis, MS

To all who are affected every hour of every day with diabetes: to those concerned with when the next low-blood-sugar event will occur; to those worried about future complications of diabetes, including blindness, amputation, kidney failure, heart disease, and premature death; and to those who will need ever-increasing medications at ever-increasing costs on their current high-carbohydrate diets. The information presented here has given many of my patients (and me) a new lease on life. It is my sincere hope that you will experience all the benefits that my patients have reported and that I am now enjoying: reduction or elimination of hypoglycemia, hyperglycemia, and diabetic complications, along with an improvement in blood sugars and a reduction in medications.

And to my parents, Barbara Z. Runyan and John W. Runyan Jr., who have supported me my entire life and therefore made this book possible.

Keith R. Runyan, MS, MD

Contents

Using This Book

Here are some tips on getting the most out of this book.

- Do yourself a favor: Read this entire book carefully. Don't skim it or skip pages. Although we welcome questions, individuals have written to us about suffering side effects that could have been avoided by reading the book carefully and in its entirety.

- In the References section, we have included a glossary of terms and endnotes which list studies that support the statements in this book. The endnotes are designated throughout the book by number.

- Additional information and more technical discussions on various topics are discussed in Tech Notes, which are available at no charge upon request. These notes are supplemental information and are offered for those who appreciate learning more about the science and medicine of diabetes. If you are that type of person, please let us know, and we will email you a PDF of the information, or you can download the file from this URL: http://www.ketogenic-diet-resource.com/support-files/ct2d-kd-tn.pdf.

Introduction

This book is designed to introduce to you an underutilized but well-researched form of treatment for diabetes, the ketogenic diet. This is not a new "fad" diet. It was first devised by Dr. John Rollo in 1797. Clinical studies of its use were published in 1921, prior to the discovery of insulin that same year.[1] The discovery of insulin in 1921 was considered "the cure" for diabetes, and dietary therapies were no longer promoted.

Our goal is to help you understand why current methods of diabetes treatment, which use a high-carbohydrate diet, medications and insulin, are ineffective by comparison. The ketogenic diet is a powerful tool for normalizing blood sugar (blood glucose). It can minimize costly and disabling long-term complications of diabetes while simultaneously minimizing hypoglycemia (low blood sugar). As a bonus, following the diet can reduce insulin and medication requirements, which not only reduce the cost of caring for diabetes but also reduce the potential for side effects.

In working with your physician and learning how to manage diabetes with a ketogenic diet, you will be able to control your blood sugar more effectively with less medication or insulin. In addition, your success in improving blood-sugar control and minimizing hypoglycemia may convince your physician to share this highly effective treatment with their other diabetic patients.

As with any diabetes treatment, the ketogenic diet needs to be combined with close monitoring of blood sugar. Urine and/or blood ketones may also require monitoring at times, and insulin dosages and other medications may need to be adjusted to maintain normal blood-glucose levels. Better blood-sugar control, fewer episodes of hypoglycemia, and a reduction in the complications of diabetes are the rewards for those who are willing to faithfully follow a ketogenic diet.

As a type 1 diabetic and a physician specializing in internal medicine, Dr. Runyan draws from both his personal experience and his clinical experience with the ketogenic diet in the treatment of diabetes in adults. He has personally witnessed many patients realize a drastic reduction in or a discontinuation of their medication or insulin requirements after putting them on the diet.

We are aware that the ketogenic diet goes against conventional wisdom. Should you decide to adopt this lifestyle, you may receive cautionary warnings from your friends, your family, or even your doctor—warnings like "All that fat will clog your arteries!" or "You need 130 grams of carbohydrate per day to fuel your brain," or "Your cholesterol will increase, and that's bad for your heart." You get the picture. We will attempt to dispel these and other myths regarding a ketogenic diet.

The stakes are high. Never underestimate the adverse consequences of elevated blood sugars and frequent or severe low blood sugars. Dr. Runyan has spent a career treating diabetic complications, including end-stage kidney failure as a result of diabetic nephropathy. He has also seen patients in a permanent comatose state from anoxic brain injury due to prolonged severe hypoglycemia. Equally sad, he knows of two young type 1 diabetic resident physicians who died of hypoglycemia while on duty at the hospital. Thousands of people suffer tragic diabetic events in the United States each year.[2] Many of these events are avoidable if people have the knowledge and the will to carefully follow the suggestions contained in this book under their physician's supervision.

Finally, we acknowledge that the ketogenic diet is not necessarily the best nor the optimal diet for all people. If, after consultation with your physician or other professional advisors knowledgeable in the ketogenic diet, you are not realizing improvements or find that the ketogenic lifestyle is not enjoyable or otherwise not right for you, please adjust the diet or find another approach to treating your diabetes. Where there's a will, there's a way—you just need to find yours.

Preface

Hello and welcome! My name is Ellen Davis, and I am the author of Ketogenic Diet Resource, a website which showcases how a ketogenic diet can be used to improve many disease conditions, and in particular, all forms of diabetes. Utilizing a ketogenic diet can help those with diabetes control their blood sugar much more easily and effectively, which means they will be able to enjoy a much improved quality of life, and avoid the menace of diabetic complications in the future.

My coauthor, Dr. Keith Runyan, is a retired physician who has type 1 diabetes, so he has intimate knowledge about effective management of this disease. His personal story in chapter 1 is a powerful testament to the benefits that people with diabetes can expect when adopting a ketogenic diet.

Although I have a master of science degree in applied clinical nutrition and Dr. Runyan is a physician, we both recommend that your personal physician be involved in the review and application of information in this book. This dietary change has a powerful effect on the body, and the dosages of blood-sugar-lowering medication and insulin will typically need to be reduced from the start of the diet. The same goes for other medications, such as those for lowering blood pressure.

I've learned over the years that each day offers a new opportunity for improved health, and it's never too late to take better care of yourself. I hope the information in this book will help you achieve that objective.

Ellen Davis, MS

Hello, my name is Keith Runyan, and I'm a retired physician who practiced internal medicine, nephrology, and obesity medicine in St. Petersburg, Florida. I attended medical school at Emory University School of Medicine in Atlanta, Georgia. Upon graduation from medical school in 1986, I completed my internship and residency in internal medicine at the Emory University Affiliated Hospitals Program. I decided to sub-specialize in nephrology, which deals with the diagnosis and treatment of kidney diseases and the treatment of kidney failure with dialysis and kidney transplantation. I am board certified in internal medicine and nephrology by the American Board of Internal Medicine and in obesity medicine by the American Board of Obesity Medicine.

In 1998, I was diagnosed with type 1 diabetes, also called latent autoimmune diabetes in adults (LADA). I treated my diabetes as recommended by the American Diabetes Association (ADA). Although my HbA1c values (a measure of average blood sugar) were in the recommended range, they were not normal, which put me at risk for diabetic complications. In addition, I was having two to five low-blood-sugar episodes each week, which was both miserable and life-threatening. I found the solution to these problems: the ketogenic diet.

After adopting the diet in February 2012, I found that my hypoglycemia was markedly reduced and my blood-sugar control was much improved. I feel obligated to convey this information to others who are willing to receive it. This is the reason for writing this book. My coauthor, Ellen Davis, has a different story but found the same solution in the ketogenic diet, and we have teamed up as advocates for this lifestyle.

Keith Runyan, MS, MD

Part 1

Setting the Stage

1

Power of the Ketogenic Diet: Personal Stories

We think real results are of great interest to all. Here are a few accounts of people who have used a ketogenic diet to improve their type 1 or type 2 diabetic-health outcomes in powerful ways.

These stories highlight several important points. First, they show how dietary changes can have powerful effects on diabetic-health outcomes—an improvement over relying solely on diabetic drugs. And, second, even though there are many well-designed studies that show that a ketogenic diet is the most effective method for lowering blood sugar, many physicians still don't know about it, and the American Diabetes Association still does not endorse it. We find this puzzling and frustrating, to say the least, and it's part of the reason for creating this book.

Keith R. Runyan, MS, MD

In 1998, at the age of thirty-eight, I was diagnosed with type 1 diabetes, also called latent autoimmune diabetes in adults (LADA). Once the diagnosis was made, I treated my diabetes with multiple insulin injections and frequent blood-sugar monitoring with the advice of endocrinologists along the way. Neither I nor my endocrinologists gave any thought to a change in diet since I was already following a "healthy" dietary regimen as recommended by the American Diabetes

Association. We were pleased that my hemoglobin A1c (HbA1c) tests were hovering between 6.5% and 7% most of the time. Although my HbA1c values were in the ADA-recommended range for diabetics (6.5%–7%), they were certainly not in the normal range for non-diabetics (which is something closer to 4.2%–5.6%). With those values, there was no assurance that I would not develop long-term diabetic complications at some point.

I was having two to five hypoglycemic episodes each week, which I thought were just part of having fairly well-controlled diabetes. My hypoglycemic symptoms ranged from clothes-soaking sweats, rapid and pounding heartbeats, blurred or double vision, transient numbness of skin, and many other symptoms that varied from episode to episode. The most bothersome were the mental symptoms of hypoglycemia. These included an inability to recognize that I was hypoglycemic—therefore, I was not aware that I needed to treat it. This also manifested itself as being argumentative with my family when they told me to take sugar when I felt I did not need any.

Hypoglycemia was an embarrassing event since it meant a lack of control, and it was worsened by the fact that I am a physician and should have all the resources and knowledge to avoid it. More importantly, hypoglycemia can be life-threatening, and, although I never lost consciousness, had a seizure, needed assistance, or had to be hospitalized, there was no assurance that any of those things would not happen while I was treating my diabetes using conventional therapy.

I was constantly thinking about how I was feeling and if how I felt could be yet another symptom of hypoglycemia. While lying down to sleep, I wondered whether I would wake up in the night in a sweat from yet another episode of low blood sugar—or not wake up at all! There was a three to four-month period when my glucose meter was unknowingly reading falsely high. This caused me to overdose insulin, which resulted in nightmarish hypoglycemic episodes so severe that I felt I might die. Fortunately, I was able to manage them myself without needing assistance. I finally purchased a new glucose meter, which put an end to the death-defying episodes. After those experiences, I checked the meter reading against laboratory glucose results, purchased new meters on a more regular basis, and sought out the most accurate meters to purchase.

What I didn't know then was that controlling diabetes with the ADA's high-carbohydrate diet without having recurrent hypoglycemia is impossible. After all, who would have imagined that respected diabetes experts would recommend an impossible task? Do you think I'm still angry? You bet. Having recurrent symptomatic hypoglycemia is certainly not a good way to go through life, especially since it can be avoided!

In August 2007, at the age of forty-seven, I decided to start exercising; I knew I had a chronic disease that might be helped by regular exercise. I decided to start training regularly to complete a sprint triathlon: a 0.9-mile swim, a 10-mile bike ride, and a 3.1-mile run. Having a goal provided additional motivation for me. I completed my first sprint-distance triathlon in December 2007. After a few years of increasing the distance of the triathlon events, I contemplated doing the full iron-man distance triathlon. I started looking into how to keep my body fueled and my blood sugars near normal for the duration of the event, particularly since sugar is the primary fuel used by most athletes during a long-distance triathlon. I was consuming sugar in order to prevent hypoglycemia to the point that I was having hyperglycemia (high blood sugars) more often than not. My HbA1c, a test of average blood sugar over time, had increased to as high as 7.9% as a result, and I feared that it would reverse any benefit of exercise.

In 2011, I signed up to enter an iron-man distance triathlon that consisted of a 2.4-mile swim, a 112-mile bike ride, and a 26.2-mile marathon run. Due to my frequent hyperglycemia while consuming sugar, and the constant threat of hypoglycemia, I felt I needed a new approach. That same year, I was listening to a triathlon podcast, *IM Talk*, hosted by John Newsom and Bevan James Eyles, in which they interviewed Loren Cordain, PhD. That interview introduced me to the concept of diseases of Western civilization. Briefly stated, people who have never been exposed to foods created by agriculture and technology (mainly highly refined sugars and starches, including sweets, flour, white rice, and fruit preserves) rarely develop chronic diseases like dental caries, diabetes, hypertension, heart disease, obesity, dementia, cancer, appendicitis, and peptic ulcers. As a physician, this came as quite a shock to me. One would think that physicians who spend their entire careers treating these chronic diseases would have been taught this in medical school. Soon after, I heard Jimmy Moore's "Livin' la Vida Low Carb" podcast interview with Dr. Richard K. Bernstein, a diabetes specialist in New York who also had type 1 diabetes. After obtaining one of the first blood-glucose meters available, he discovered by trial and error that carbohydrates had the greatest influence on his blood sugars and that a ketogenic diet containing less than 30 grams carbohydrate per day normalized his blood-sugar levels with a much-reduced insulin dosage.

From the tenets of *The Paleo Diet*, as described by Dr. Cordain, I placed more emphasis on using real whole foods and paid more attention to the source of foods. I added grass-fed beef; free-range, pastured chicken; pork; liver; and wild fish to my diet. One can have success with conventionally sourced foods, but I appreciated some of the significant differences that grass-fed and pastured foods had to offer.

Still skeptical that conventional medicine could possibly be so wrong, I was on a mission to both verify what Dr. Cordain was saying and to learn more about how nutrition affects health and disease. I read Gary Taubes's book *Good Calories, Bad Calories* on the history of diseases of Western civilization, the origin of the low-fat diet, lipid-heart and carbohydrate hypotheses, and the evidence supporting the role of dietary refined carbohydrates and sugar in the causation of chronic diseases. I read Dr. Bernstein's *Diabetes Solution*, which described his method of using the ketogenic diet to treat diabetes, and many other books and articles, including many cited in this book. I wanted to make sure that the information I was obtaining was accurate since

I was changing my own treatment in opposition to current medical convention.

I also utilized information from *The Art and Science of Low Carbohydrate Living* and *The Art and Science of Low Carbohydrate Performance* by Stephen Phinney, MD, PhD, and Jeff Volek, PhD, RD. When I learned that their information was accurate, I became angry. Why had I not taken the initiative to find this out for myself sooner? Why didn't the world's leading diabetes experts and organizations find this out or mention it as an option? Why didn't the research-funding organizations support studies to test the carbohydrate hypothesis? How could so many scientists and physicians come to believe that a diet with six to eleven daily servings of bread, cereal, rice, and pasta was a "healthy" diet, especially for people with diabetes? After all, those people are the most intolerant of high-carbohydrate foods. In addition, the practice of consuming large amounts of refined foods never existed on the planet until a few hundred years ago. How could humans adapt to them in such a short time on the evolutionary time scale?

So, on February 8, 2012, I started my new lifestyle: a ketogenic diet added to the resistance training, swimming, biking, and running that I had started in 2007. From what I learned reading *The Paleo Diet*, I had already eliminated milk, grains, sugar, starchy legumes, and all processed foods in November 2011.

Following *The Paleo Diet* plan led to a 45% reduction in my mealtime insulin dose but no improvement in my average blood sugar nor any reduction in hypoglycemic episodes. I needed carbohydrate restriction added to the mix. In order to reduce my carbohydrate intake to 25 to 35 grams per day, I eliminated potatoes and fruit except for a few occasional strawberries or blueberries. To replace calories from the carbohydrates that I eliminated, I increased my dietary fat using small amounts of coconut and olive oils and butter. I simultaneously reduced my insulin doses (both long-acting and short-acting insulins) from about fifty-four units a day to about thirty-five units a day over the next month or so, but I continued to adjust the insulin dose based on my blood-sugar readings and exercise. The variables I tracked included insulin doses, exercise type and duration, and fat intake based on appetite and energy expenditure. The constants I sought to maintain included the ketogenic diet with moderate-protein and low-carbohydrate intake, keeping my blood sugar as close to normal as I could safely accomplish, i.e., avoiding hypoglycemia.

Once I adapted to the ketogenic diet, I was able to increase my training distances without needing to eat significant amounts of sugar. I developed the habit of carrying both insulin and glucose tablets with me, just in case, but I rarely needed either of them. I no longer feared hypoglycemia, even while exercising, and my hyperglycemia improved markedly.

On October 20, 2012, I completed the Great Floridian Triathlon, an iron-man distance event, in fifteen and a half hours with no need for any glucose, sugar, or food, using only my body-fat reserves for energy. I had no hypoglycemia, but I did have mild hyperglycemia that I did not treat with insulin because I was expecting my blood sugar to fall at some point during the event. My blood sugar at the end of the event was 156 mg/dL.

My HbA1c improved gradually, from 6.5% on average before the ketogenic diet, to 5.6% in the first year on the ketogenic diet. In 2013, it remained at 5.6% and, in 2014, came down to 5.1% with an average blood glucose of 85 mg/dL. This resulted in more hypoglycemia, albeit without symptoms (more on that later); subsequently, I have accepted a near-normal blood glucose—around 95 mg/dL—in exchange for fewer hypoglycemic episodes.

My blood tests have improved in the manner typically seen on a ketogenic diet. Triglycerides decreased from an average of 76 to 65 mg/dL; HDL cholesterol increased from an average of 61 to 90 mg/dL; the triglyceride/HDL ratio decreased from 1.31 to 0.72; and the calculated LDL cholesterol increased from an average of 103 to 162 mg/dL but later came down to 132 mg/dL. The hs-CRP (high-sensitivity C-reactive protein, a marker of inflammation) decreased from 3.2 to

0.7 mg/L. I have chronicled my personal results on my blog: http:// ketogenicdiabeticathlete.wordpress.com.

Today, I have no complications from diabetes, and, with my improved glycemic control, my outlook on life has improved dramatically.

Carl Martin

Men's Health did a story on me once, then they never published it. Guess they were worried about sponsors. The story was about how I controlled my diabetes with diet and exercise and no meds.

I am sure I had diabetes for at least a decade before diagnosing myself approximately fifteen years ago. I was getting physicals from my doctor every year, but my blood glucose was never checked. I got very sick; I was seriously ill. I had all the classic symptoms, so I went to my doctor and told him I had diabetes. There was no good advice from him, only prescriptions for drugs to take. I have had many doctors over the years and have received no good advice from any of them. No doctor ever told me the most important thing I needed to do—lose weight and cut the carbs out of my diet.

A friend of mine who was also diabetic gave me the best advice I ever got from anyone about how to control my diabetes. He told me to lose fifty pounds, and the symptoms would go away. I went on the late great Dr. Robert Atkins diet. I lost eighty-five pounds, and the symptoms did go away. I was always a bicycle commuter and got plenty of exercise. I would say extreme exercise. Exercise alone is not enough. It has to be diet and exercise to be effective. I have always ridden a bicycle twenty miles a day commuting to work. One of the first things I learned was that I had to take control of my own health. Doctors never provided me with anything positive about controlling my health. My very best source of information came from David Mendosa's diabetic website. David is fabulous. I also have been friends over the web with Jimmy Moore since he started his blog.

Over the years, the weight would come back, and I would look for ways to be able to eat a more normal diet—the magic pill. I tried all the new latest medications: Byetta, Januvia, Victosa, and many others; I finally started Lantus insulin. They all were effective for a while but not for long. The blood sugar would start creeping up. The drugs would initially work but not for long. The drugs all stopped working. Insulin stopped working. I did not like taking insulin. I know how damaging it was to my body.

My weight was going up, but, more importantly, my blood sugar was going way up. So I went back on my ketogenic diet. My blood sugar instantly dropped to normal, even below normal, I never expected such dramatic results, even though I had years of experience with low-carb diets. I have been off insulin for a while now and have never had better blood-glucose levels. My weight is slowly going down, and I have pulled a notch in my belt. Naturally, I feel better. I should have been most worried about my health, but I was also determined that I was not going to buy larger-size clothes!

I ran across Ellen's site and think it is excellent. I am amazed how much great information is now available on the Internet. When I first discovered I had diabetes, about the only good information I could find on the web was from David Mendosa and Jimmy Moore. David and I took the same journey with diabetic control. We started Byetta at the same time, when it was new. David dropped the drugs and went to very low-carb eating and cured his diabetes.

Clair Schwan

Having been diagnosed several years ago with type 2 diabetes, my doctor recommended Metformin as a course of treatment, along with vigorous exercise and a diet emphasizing complex carbohydrates. I generally went along with the diet and exercise recommendations but insisted that I wasn't going to use any medication to address my higher-than-normal fasting blood-glucose readings. After all, I wasn't a flaming diabetic with blood-sugar readings in the 200 to 300 range, but rather in the low 100s. I figured that I ought to be able to fix this on my own. I also considered that if I were to use medication as a crutch,

I might needlessly create a dependency on medication for a condition that I essentially gave to myself through my own neglect. I thought it was entirely possible to rid myself of this condition by simply being a better caretaker of me.

As a first step, I generally followed a low-carbohydrate diet, but I wasn't doing anything precise or scientific. Nevertheless, the results were encouraging. My fasting blood sugars were in the high normal to pre-diabetic range, typically 91 to 118. Based on these preliminary trials, my physician confirmed that my condition was indeed reversible, if only I paid closer attention to diet and exercise.

After learning more about a special type of low-carbohydrate diet, known as a ketogenic diet, I began to understand more about the science behind it, and I started to appreciate that implementation had to be done with some level of precision in order to be effective. My blood sugars were stubbornly in the pre-diabetic range, while all the rest of my blood work was normal. So, the time had come to apply a more scientific approach to my diet.

I undertook a twenty-three-day application of the ketogenic diet as a trial, with strict application of criteria for fat, protein, and carbohydrate intake. As a result, my fasting blood sugar dropped a total of 53 points, from a high of 125 to a low of 72. A normal fasting blood-sugar reading of 88 was achieved on day six of the diet, and during the last two weeks of the trial, my average morning blood-sugar reading was 86. In addition to a reduction in fasting blood sugars, I lost a much needed twenty-two pounds and had to cut back my blood-pressure medications to one quarter the dosage because my blood pressure was significantly lower as well. All of this occurred simply because of a change in diet; I didn't do anything special in terms of exercise.

During my trial application, I learned many things about the ketogenic diet that are important. First, although the percentage of fat intake is relatively high when compared with protein and carbohydrate, since fat has more than twice the calories per gram, it's relatively easy to meet fat requirements by simply going a bit heavy on butter and bacon grease when preparing meals. Second, it's clear that fat doesn't make you fat; instead, it's a great alternate fuel to replace the glucose that most of us are conditioned to use. Third, keeping protein at a modest level prevents conversion of excess protein to glucose during gluconeogenesis, which occurs while you sleep. Fourth, even raw carrots cause a considerable increase in fasting blood-sugar readings, so I now avoid them. Fifth, after a couple of weeks on the diet, hunger seems to disappear, and that makes staying on the diet much easier.

Based on what I've seen, heard, read, and experienced, it's clear to me that no single formula for lowering and stabilizing blood sugars will work for everyone. Nevertheless, the ketogenic diet has many clear benefits to offer to those of us who are carbohydrate intolerant. It will be an important tool in my health-care toolbox from now on.

Carsten Thomsen

Hello. My name is Carsten, and December 13, 1975, is when my long journey dealing with type 1 diabetes began. On December 12, I had eaten an entire large pizza, a box of fried chicken, and a half-gallon of ice cream. After consuming all that food, I lost five pounds while sleeping.

My parents immediately took me to the doctor to have me checked out. When my blood sugar was tested, and the result was 425, it was pretty easy for the doctor to make his diagnosis: I had type 1 juvenile diabetes mellitus.

I was sent to see a dietician to fill me in on how I should be eating as a type 1 diabetic. I was told to eat the proper amount of food by weighing all of my portions, to eat very little fat or protein, and to eat lots of fruits and carbohydrates.

For the next ten years, I tried my best to follow the standard recommendations for keeping my blood sugar under control. I ate what they told me to eat (standard American Diabetes Association recommendations), exercised when I could, and kept taking my insulin shots.

The problem was that I kept gaining weight, I was always tired, and I was taking huge amounts of insulin.

Looking back on that diet now, I'm surprised that I'm not dead.

I followed that plan for a long time. I constantly fought weight gain and could barely keep my blood-sugar levels under control. At the time, I was taking one hundred units of insulin a day. For those of you who don't take insulin, one hundred units is a major amount. Over a period of time, I also gained thirty-five pounds.

I've worked in the health profession as an environmental health specialist for the last thirty years. My career has enabled me to keep close track of information related to medical conditions, nutrition, and the effects of the environment on health. About twenty-five years ago, I discovered that the traditional way I was taught to control my diabetes was certainly not the only way. I've spent thousands of hours doing research on what I could do to live a healthier life. I took the best available knowledge and applied it to myself.

During my research, I found a few diabetes specialists who were promoting a totally different approach by controlling diabetes with diet. These specialists evaluated medical information on how diabetics were treated before insulin was available. Before insulin treatment, diabetes was treated by eating meals consisting mostly of fats, with some proteins and low-carbohydrate vegetables, which controlled the blood-sugar levels.

After reading the research, the experiences I was having with a high-carbohydrate diet made a lot of sense to me. I decided to eat large amounts of fat, small amounts of protein, and some low-carbohydrate vegetables. After following that diet for several months, I was amazed at the results.

By removing almost all of the carbohydrates from my diet, my blood-sugar levels became very stable. I was not hungry all the time, and, best of all, the amount of insulin I needed dropped by almost 80%. I was excited with my results, and I wanted to share them with my doctor. I told him about the diet I was using, and he had a fit. He informed me that if I continued eating all that fat and protein I would become obese and probably die of a heart attack or kidney disease.

I was feeling so good though, and I persisted with my newfound diet. To be cautious and make sure I wasn't hurting myself, I had my cholesterol, triglycerides, and kidney-function levels checked frequently. To my doctor's subdued amazement, my overall cholesterol level dropped, my good (HDL) cholesterol level increased, my triglyceride level dropped like a rock, and my kidney-function levels did not change at all. I've now been on this diet for about twenty years, and all of my blood markers and kidney-function levels have continued in the "very healthy" ranges.

I hope I have conveyed to you through this brief story about my life with diabetes how much better I feel and how much healthier I am after cutting out all those carbohydrates from my diet. I'm sure not everybody will have the same results I've had through my journey, but I've been totally blessed with minimal impact on my health—even after forty years of being a type 1 diabetic. I urge anyone who has type 1 or type 2 diabetes to give a low-carbohydrate, high-fat diet a chance. By doing so, your overall health can be changed in wonderful, amazing ways.

Sandy Bahr

I was diagnosed with type 2 diabetes in December 2009, with blood sugars from the 180s to the 220s (10–12.3 mmol) and an A1c of 8.6. It was certainly not unexpected, given my family history and my gestational diabetes during my pregnancies.

When I went to my first diabetes education class, I was the only newly diagnosed diabetic there who was not on medication yet (thanks to a doctor who believed in me). That was my last diabetes education class. The idea of eating corn flakes and sugar-laden low-fat yogurt just struck me as wrong. It has been a journey—and a lot of trial and error!

I went pretty much grain free and low carb in 2011, but I still couldn't get my morning blood sugar down, and my after-meal blood sugar was 130 to 140 mg/dL. This was not acceptable to me as I remembered reading in Dr. Bernstein's book that blood sugars over 130 would continue to cause organ damage.

In December of 2012, I read the book *The Art & Science of Low Carbohydrate Living* by Stephen Phinney and Jeff Volek. It has become my diabetes bible. I began the ketogenic diet program described in their book, and a miracle took place in my life. Within five days, my blood sugars normalized, and I was seeing a fasting blood sugar under 100 and after-meal blood sugars in the 90s. I was pinching myself in disbelief!

I had my yearly "preventative" exam in January 2015, after twenty-six months on the ketogenic diet. I say that because I no longer have to have diabetes follow-up exams. My doctor has declared me to be no longer diabetic "on paper" (as she says). She was completely blown away by my labs and could hardly believe my numbers:

- Fasting blood glucose on day of testing was 74 (4.1 mmol), and HbA1c was 5.3.
- Homocysteine was down to 9.8 from 11.8 in 2013. This is a marker for heart disease. Below 10 is fine. Over 13 or so is concerning.

All of my liver enzymes were improved over the previous three years. So much for the propaganda saying that a high-fat diet causes fatty liver!

My total cholesterol of 222 was borderline, but it was higher due to the higher "healthy" HDL. My LDL of 106 was near optimal (down from 144), and my HDL of 92 was optimal (up 40 points from last year). More importantly, my triglyceride level of 120 was normal (145 last year). My ratios improved as well:

- Total cholesterol/HDL ratio (preferably <5.0, ideally <3.5) was 2.41—ideal.
- LDL/HDL ratio (preferably <5.0, ideally <2.0) was 1.152—ideal.
- Triglycerides/HDL ratio (preferably <4, ideally <2) was 1.304—ideal.

I "teach" the ketogenic diet for use in diabetes in two Facebook groups, and many more are now finding the same success that I have found. You can find my personal blog at http://ketodiabetes.blogspot.com.

2

Ketogenic Diets and Diabetes

Now that we've shared some personal success stories, let's explore some specific information on how ketogenic diets work, how diabetes works, and how ketogenic diets can improve diabetic health outcomes.

What Is a Ketogenic Diet?

All diets consist of three key macronutrients: fats, such as butter and oil; carbohydrates, found in sweets and starchy foods; and protein, found in meats, dairy and nuts. A ketogenic diet is high in fat, moderate in protein, and very low in carbohydrate.

A ketogenic diet restricts carbohydrate intake to about 2% to 10% of total calories. In contrast, the US Department of Agriculture (USDA) guidelines for a standard American diet (SAD) recommend that 45% to 65% of calories come from carbohydrates, the nutrient to which a person with diabetes is most intolerant.

The difference between these two diets is in their cellular-fuel effects. The high quantities of carbohydrate-containing foods consumed on the SAD are broken down into large amounts of blood sugar. This, in turn, causes a rise in the need for insulin, a hormone that acts to push sugar from the bloodstream into our cells where it can be stored or broken down into energy for the body. The more carbohydrates eaten, the more insulin is needed to deal with the resulting elevations in blood glucose.

In contrast, when carbohydrate intake is restricted and protein intake is moderate, blood glucose and insulin needs are reduced, and this causes a biochemical adaptation and shift toward the use of fat instead of glucose to fuel body cells. As a result, stored fat is more easily liberated from fat tissue, and there is an increase in ketogenesis, a process in which the liver creates ketone bodies from fatty acids and releases them into the bloodstream so that the brain, muscles, and other tissues can use them as an alternate fuel. Ketone bodies are metabolic byproducts that result when the body shifts fuel sources and burns fat more readily than carbohydrates. We are accustomed to hearing that carbohydrates are the body's preferred fuel, but the truth is, the human body is capable of thriving on fats and ketones.

The two to three-week process of restricting carbohydrates to increase fat and ketone-producing enzymes is called fat-adaptation and keto-adaptation. Once the body is "keto-adapted" and has made the switch from using glucose to using fat and ketones as the primary fuel, that person is said to be in "nutritional ketosis." Ketosis is an evolutionary adaptation to food scarcity.[3] In fact, the biochemical effect of a ketogenic diet is very similar to the effect of a complete fast from food. When food is unavailable, the most crucial task of the body's energy systems is to provide glucose to fuel the brain. No glucose for the brain equates to no life. In addition, muscle mass has to be protected so that a hunt for food can continue. Ketosis is the perfect solution. Once keto-adapted, the body uses fatty acids and ketones from stored fat to fuel most cells, and glucose needs are reduced. Otherwise, if the body were to continue to depend on glucose alone, most of the muscle tissue would be quickly consumed. This is because during prolonged food deprivation, muscle is broken down into its amino-acid building blocks, which are then converted to glucose for the brain.

In addition, there are some profound and positive health effects[4] when the body uses ketones as its primary fuel source. For instance, cellular inflammation and free-radical activity are reduced. There is also less glycation damage. Glycation and free-radical activity contribute to the development and progression of a long list of diabetic complications, including kidney damage,[5] blindness,[6] peripheral nerve damage,[7] and heart disease.[8] It's not such a leap in logic to consider that our bodies are meant to run on ketones, given the positive health effects they bestow.

The antioxidant and anti-inflammatory effects of nutritional ketosis are why calorie restriction, fasting, and ketogenic diets have such beneficial effects on human health. In fact, nutritional ketosis and ketone bodies themselves are being studied extensively as a treatment for many metabolic diseases. A growing number of research papers[9] have been published on the anti-inflammatory effect of ketones on conditions such as epilepsy, multiple sclerosis, ALS, Parkinson's disease, Alzheimer's disease, head trauma, cancer, cardiovascular disease, autism, migraine headaches, stroke, depression, acne, and, of course, diabetes.[10]

The takeaway here is that the ketogenic diet is not a fad. It is a potent regulator of metabolic derangement, and, when formulated and implemented correctly, it can be extremely effective, especially in the treatment of diabetes.

What Is Diabetes?

Diabetes is a group of diseases that are characterized by high levels of glucose or sugar in the bloodstream resulting from either a lack of insulin or dysfunctional insulin signaling. According to the American Diabetes Association's 2014 National Report,[11] over twenty-one million Americans were diagnosed with diabetes, and another eight million have diabetes but remain undiagnosed; these numbers are predicted to increase dramatically in the future. People with uncontrolled diabetes develop serious complications leading to heart disease, stroke, kidney failure, amputations, blindness, and death.

There are several different types of diabetes.[12] Type 1 diabetes mellitus (T1DM) and type 2 diabetes mellitus (T2DM) are the most common. T1DM is an autoimmune disease that primarily affects children, adolescents, and young adults. If it occurs in adults, it is designated as latent autoimmune diabetes in adults (LADA). In contrast, T2DM primarily affects adults, but the rates of this disease are escalating in younger adults, adolescents, and children. Eighty-five percent of people with T2DM are overweight or obese. The cause of T2DM is severe insulin resistance (resistance to the effect of insulin), which can first manifest as metabolic syndrome and prediabetes. The list below shows pertinent differences between types of diabetes.

Type 1 Diabetes

- Affects children and adolescents
- Autoimmune disease
- Pancreatic beta cells non-functional; no insulin secreted
- Insulin must be injected
- 5%–10% of all diabetes diagnoses

LADA (Latent Autoimmune Diabetes in Adults)

- Affects young adults to elderly
- Autoimmune disease
- Slower destruction of pancreatic beta cells
- Pancreatic beta cells non-functional; no insulin secreted
- Insulin must be injected

Type 2 Diabetes

- Can strike at any age
- Insulin resistance is the defining disease factor
- Obesity is a symptom
- Pancreatic beta cells functional; insulin secreted, sometimes in large amounts
- Non-insulin dependent (but may need insulin to control blood sugar)

Although type 1 diabetes (T1DM) results from the autoimmune destruction of the beta cells and the loss of both insulin and amylin secretion, type 2 diabetes (T2DM) is a multisystem disorder that begins with the development of insulin resistance in multiple tissues, including muscle, liver, and adipose tissue, with secondary hyperinsulinemia (excess insulin secretion into the blood), and only in the late stage of the disease does insulin secretion become impaired.

The beta cells are part of a structure called the islet of Langerhans in the pancreas. Insulin and amylin, the hormones that beta cells secrete, regulate the neighboring alpha cells, which secrete a hormone called glucagon, and the delta cells, which produce a hormone called somatostatin. Somatostatin can inhibit both insulin and glucagon secretion. Together, the beta cells, alpha cells, and delta cells carefully regulate blood glucose and regulate metabolism throughout the body. When the beta cells become dysfunctional or are destroyed, this elegant regulation is lost, resulting in the symptoms of diabetes.

Insulin is a key hormone that controls not only blood glucose but also many other aspects of fuel metabolism. Insulin's main function is to transfer glucose from the blood into body cells so that it can be metabolized for energy or stored as glycogen, a larger molecule found primarily in the liver and skeletal muscle. For people with a fully functioning pancreas, this transfer and storage process happens when food is ingested and metabolized. It may take several hours for all food to be broken down and absorbed. Once all of the incoming food is stored or metabolized for energy, insulin has completed its job and blood-sugar levels begin to drop.

If the next meal is skipped or delayed, the alpha cells of the pancreas secrete glucagon. Glucagon signals the liver to break down stored glycogen into glucose and release it into the blood to maintain normal blood-sugar levels. The liver may also produce glucose from various "precursor" molecules in a process called gluconeogenesis. In addition, fatty acids may be produced for fuel as the rate of ketogenesis increases.

Diabetes is diagnosed when blood-sugar levels rise above normal, either because the pancreas is damaged by an autoimmune attack and stops making insulin, as in type 1 diabetes, or because the body

nsitive to insulin's message (insulin resistance), as in type
he symptoms of diabetes include the following:

- Polyuria (frequent urination)
- Polydipsia (drinking lots of fluids)
- Thirst and dry mouth
- Extreme fatigue
- Blurry vision
- Cuts and bruises that are slow to heal
- Tingling, pain, or numbness in the hands and feet
- Hunger, weight loss

The danger of diabetes is in the lack of insulin or resistance to insulin that results in a blood-sugar "roller coaster" effect. High blood sugar (hyperglycemia) contributes to glycation damage and long-term complications, and low blood sugar (hypoglycemia) can cause a loss of consciousness or death if the brain runs out of fuel. In the next section, we'll explore these conditions in more detail.

Blood Glucose, Hyperglycemia and Hypoglycemia

As we learned earlier, glucose is a simple sugar that your cells use to make energy. It's created from the breakdown or metabolism of foods that contain carbohydrate (starches and sugars) and, to a lesser extent, protein foods such as meat and eggs. Glucose is utilized in the body through the action of insulin, a hormone that "pushes" glucose into body cells so it can be used to make adenosine triphosphate (ATP), the energy currency of the human body.

Blood glucose is a measure of the amount of glucose (sugar) in your bloodstream at any one time. Normally, the human body has mechanisms in place to maintain the amount of glucose in the bloodstream in a very narrow range. At any one time, normal blood sugar amounts to a little less than 5 grams[13] or one teaspoon of sugar. Mathematically, this works out to a range of about 83–99 mg/dL, the "normal" range of blood sugar.

For people with diabetes, blood-sugar levels are constantly out of the normal range. Most of the time, blood glucose is too high, a condition known as hyperglycemia. A diabetic with uncontrolled blood sugars may have two to ten times the normal amount of blood glucose. Hyperglycemia is responsible for most of the damage that results in long-term diabetic complications. The damage is done through a process called glycation in which blood sugar "sticks" to various body tissues, causing dysfunction. Because diabetic blood sugars are higher than normal for longer periods of time, more glycation damage is done. Glycation is measured using two tests. The first is called the hemoglobin A1C test (HbA1c), which measures glycation in red blood cells. While a finger-stick measurement of blood glucose is a snapshot of one moment in time, the HbA1c test is a longer-term measurement and can be thought of as reflecting average blood glucose over the previous two to three-month span. The second test is called a fructosamine test, which measures glycation in a blood protein called albumin over the previous two to three-week period.

Diabetics can also experience low blood sugar or hypoglycemia, and this can be even more dangerous. Without blood sugar, human body systems cease to function; in the case of the human brain, a lack of blood sugar can result in a loss of consciousness, seizures, coma, and death. Hypoglycemia is a constant danger for diabetics, especially those using insulin, a sulfonylurea, or a glinide drug to manage excess blood sugar.

In the next section, we will explore how different food choices affect blood sugar and insulin levels, and why it's important for those with diabetes to minimize carbohydrate intake.

Food Choices, Blood Sugar and Insulin

For people with diabetes, the dynamics of blood sugar and insulin are a primary focus each day. Controlling the long-term complications of diabetes is dependent upon managing insulin and its effect on blood sugar. This is why the types and amounts of foods eaten are important, and this is where a ketogenic diet makes a difference. Let's take a closer look at how food choices affect blood sugar and insulin needs.

Foods in the human diet are composed of three important macronutrients: fats, carbohydrates, and proteins. Upon digestion in the body, each of these macronutrients has a different effect on blood sugar and on insulin needs as described below.

Most dietary fats and oils are in the form of triglycerides, which can be either saturated (butter, coconut oil), monounsaturated (olive oil), or polyunsaturated (vegetable oils such as safflower or soybean). Of the three macronutrients, dietary fat has the least stimulatory effect on blood sugar. Dietary fat also slows the rate of absorption of carbohydrates and, therefore, mitigates somewhat their effect on blood glucose. The need for insulin is lower.

Proteins are primarily found in foods such as meats, eggs, poultry, fish, and some plant foods (soy, nuts, and beans). During digestion, proteins are broken down into smaller units called amino acids. Dietary protein has a moderate effect on blood sugar and requires a moderate dose of insulin. In a study by Symons et al. at the University of Texas,[14] a 113-gram protein meal increased serum insulin levels by 50%, at most.

Carbohydrates are found in foods such as dairy, fruits, vegetables, beans, grains (wheat, rice, corn), and all starchy or sweet foods. Upon digestion, carbohydrates are broken down into simple sugars (glucose, galactose, and fructose). Dietary carbohydrates have the greatest effect on blood sugar. Carbohydrates eaten in any amount or form will raise blood sugar and necessitate large doses of insulin to counteract rapid blood-sugar elevations. Large doses of insulin then increase the danger of low blood sugar.

The amount of each of these macronutrients in the diet is important as well. Fat is a structural component of all mammalian cell walls and many hormones; it also provides a major fuel source for the body. Dietary fat requirements are largely determined by body mass, total energy expenditure, and current body-fat stores. Active individuals will require more dietary fat intake, while obese individuals will require less dietary fat intake since fat already stored in the body can act as a source of energy.

Protein is primarily used as a structural and functional element in the body and is only secondarily used as a fuel. Dietary protein intake should be based on lean body mass—or goal body weight (GBW)—and the level of physical activity pursued. We will explore determining your protein needs in chapter 5.

Carbohydrates are not essential in the diet, so dietary carbohydrate intake can be based on one's carbohydrate tolerance. However, diabetes is a state of profound carbohydrate intolerance, and people with diabetes will gain the most benefit from strictly limiting dietary carbohydrates, usually to 30 to 50 grams per day.

Understanding total macronutrient intake will help you determine which foods are the best choices to increase ketosis and lower your blood sugar and insulin needs. We'll talk about customizing macronutrient intake for your individual needs later. For now, let's get back to nutritional ketosis and why it and the ketogenic diet are so helpful for people with diabetes.

Nutritional Ketosis and Your Brain

Let's explore why a ketogenic diet is better for people with diabetes. Nutritional ketosis is a metabolic state that occurs when a person either fasts or restricts carbohydrate intake. After two to three consistent weeks on a carb-restricted ketogenic diet, the liver adapts to lower glucose and insulin by producing increased quantities of ketone bodies from either dietary fat or fat released from fat cells.

Here's the important part: the liver does this because the human brain must be fueled constantly to stay alive. Any interruption in fuel availability is an emergency for the brain. And while human brains can run on both glucose and ketones, there's a balancing act involved. This issue of balanced fuel sources for the brain is crucial to understanding the positive effect of a ketogenic diet on diabetic health factors.

The crux of it is whether your brain is "carb-adapted" or "keto-adapted." Once this concept is understood, dietary choices begin to make real sense, and the benefits of a ketogenic diet for diabetes can be realized.

Is Your Brain Carb-Adapted or Keto-Adapted?

Let's explore the difference between having a brain that is carb-adapted versus having a keto-adapted brain. Carb-adapted is up first because that's typical for someone consuming a standard American diet.

When a person consumes a high-carbohydrate diet, ketone production in the liver is essentially shut off due to the presence of large amounts of circulating glucose and insulin. Since ketones are unavailable, the brain is dependent on glucose as its only fuel source. We call this a carb-adapted brain since it relies greatly on glucose to function and thrive. When a carb-adapted brain senses that blood glucose is becoming scarce (such as when food is unavailable or when too much insulin is injected), it has to take countermeasures and an adrenalin rush ensues. The adrenalin rush results in the symptoms of hypoglycemia or low blood sugar. The signal is frantic because, at this point, glucose must be made available from glucose tablets or food that is high in sugar. Otherwise, as glucose levels drop further, the carb-adapted brain can lose consciousness, and, without an intervention of glucagon by injection, glucose levels can drop to a point that results in coma or death.

For example, let's say Ben, a person with insulin-dependent type 2 diabetes, prepares a meal with a large amount of carbohydrate. Just before the meal, Ben gives himself a large injection of insulin to counteract the blood-sugar rise that he knows he will experience from the carbohydrate he eats. A few minutes into his meal, he gets a frantic phone call from a friend who needs some immediate help. Ben leaves the house in a hurry and doesn't finish his meal.

Thirty minutes later, the insulin he injected kicks in, and because he didn't eat the amount of carbohydrate he thought he would, the excess insulin drops his blood sugar to dangerously low levels. As he breaks into a sweat and starts to feel weak and dizzy, his friend realizes what is happening and gets him some orange juice to drink. This brings his blood sugar back up and offsets the effects of the excess insulin. As you can see, a frantic low-blood-sugar warning system is necessary for a carb-adapted brain.

Now consider Lisa, a type 1 diabetic who is on a ketogenic diet. Lisa restricts her carb intake to the same small amount every day. Over time, her liver has increased its ketone production. She has entered a state of "nutritional ketosis." Her blood-ketone levels stay in a range of 0.5–3 mmol/L (mM), and, at this level, the ketones can cross the blood-brain barrier and diffuse into her neurons where they can be metabolized as a fuel source. Since her brain is ketone-adapted, low blood sugar becomes less of an emergency since her brain cells now have an alternate fuel source.

Lisa is able to keep her insulin doses very small because there is no carbohydrate-induced spike in her blood sugars, and this lowers her risk of hypoglycemia. Hence, she very rarely experiences any symptoms of low blood sugar. Lisa has taken her blood sugar at times and noticed it was lower than normal, but she did not feel weak or faint. However, she made sure to correct her glucose reading to >70 mg/dL with a glucose tablet. Being keto-adapted gives her body options for keeping her brain supplied with an energy source.

In the overall evolutionary design of the human body, the ability of the liver to produce ketones is an elegant solution for protecting the brain when food is unavailable. Fasting and starvation cause the same ketone-producing effect in the body. In fact, most people wake up each morning in mild ketosis because they haven't eaten for the past eight to twelve hours. As long as dietary carbohydrate is restricted to 20 to 50 grams per day and dietary protein intake is not excessive (depending on the individual), the liver will produce ketones, and blood and urine ketone levels will rise moderately. Blood ketone levels do not typically rise as high during nutritional ketosis (0.5–3 mM) as they do during prolonged fasting (5–8 mM).

Having a keto-adapted brain is advantageous, and following a keto-genic diet bestows other benefits as well. Let's discuss some of these.

Benefits of a Ketogenic Diet

The beneficial effects of a ketogenic diet are numerous and affect many different body systems. We've discussed the most pertinent below.

> *Lower insulin doses for diabetics.* The ketogenic diet requires the least amount of insulin compared to any other diabetic dietary therapy. This explains why it's so effective in prevention and treatment of prediabetes and type 1 and type 2 diabetes. For type 2 diabetics, dietary carbohydrate restriction means the input of glucose into the bloodstream is minimized, and this places less demand on the pancreas to secrete insulin. In a 2012 Swedish study, forty-eight people with type 1 diabetes were instructed to follow a 75-gram-per-day low-carbohydrate diet. The results showed that the participants achieved a mean reduction in HbA1c from 7.6% at the start to 6.3% at just three months. After four years, the HbA1c was still only 6.9%. Mean daily mealtime insulin for thirty-six patients was reduced from 23 ± 9 IU at the start to 13 ± 6 IU at one year. Mean daily long-acting insulin was reduced modestly from 19.6 ± 5 IU to 18.6 ± 6 IU in the first year. Hypoglycemic episodes were reduced by 82%, from 2.9 to 0.5 episodes per week.[15]

> *Lower blood pressure.* Ketogenic diets are very effective at reducing blood pressure. If you are taking blood-pressure medications, be aware that this may result in feeling dizzy from too much medication. You may need to reduce your blood-pressure medication, so talk with your doctor about reassessing your medication dosage before you start.

> *Increase in HDL cholesterol and reduction in triglycerides.* In most people, following a ketogenic diet will raise HDL cholesterol while lowering triglycerides and total cholesterol.[16] This is actually a positive change because it improves the ratio of HDL to LDL.

Higher HDL levels (≥40 mg/dL (men) or ≥50 mg/dL (women)) indicate a lower risk for heart disease. Carbohydrate consumption is a direct driver of triglyceride levels in the blood. As triglycerides rise, heart-disease risks also rise. The less carbohydrate you eat, the lower your triglyceride readings will be. Triglyceride levels <100 mg/dL are achievable and optimal for persons with diabetes following a ketogenic diet.

> *Lower average blood glucose (both baseline and after meals).* As your carbohydrate intake drops, your fasting and after-meal blood sugars will drop. An average of these measurements can be seen in HbA1c test results. The HbA1c test is a long-term measure (previous two to three months) of average blood sugar. Since a ketogenic diet lowers blood sugar, HbA1c levels should drop over time.

> *Lower levels of inflammation.* The ketogenic diet is anti-inflammatory in that it reduces numerous markers of inflammation including interleukin, tumor necrosis factor-alpha, vascular endothelial growth factor, interferon-c, epidermal growth factor, monocyte chemotactic protein-1, intracellular cellular adhesion molecule-1, vascular cellular adhesion molecule-I, and nuclear factor-kappa B, as shown in a study by Forsythe et al. at the University of Connecticut.[17] A test called the high-sensitivity C-reactive protein (hs-CRP) test is used to measure total body-system inflammation. This test is also a marker for heart-disease risk, since heart disease is linked to high levels of body inflammation. An optimal hs-CRP level is < 1 mg/L. Once you start a ketogenic diet, and your blood sugar and insulin levels drop, you should see your hs-CRP level drop as well as other markers of inflammation.

> *Reduction of inappropriate hunger and sugar cravings.* Appetite is reduced on a ketogenic diet. It is not known why this occurs. It may be because fuel flow has normalized and cells are receiving adequate energy. You'll notice that, at times, you may forget to eat. You may find this is the most amazing part, especially if you struggle with food addiction.

➤ *Heartburn relief.* Some people who suffer from gastroesophageal reflux disease (GERD) or other heartburn issues notice improvement in their symptoms after starting a ketogenic diet. The results of a study at the University of North Carolina suggests that a very low-carbohydrate diet in obese individuals with GERD can significantly improve symptoms.[18]

➤ *Less gum and tooth disease.* Carbohydrate consumption feeds oral bacteria like *streptococcus mutans*, which lowers the pH of your saliva and erodes the tooth enamel, leading to tooth decay.[19] After some time on a ketogenic diet, tooth-decay issues may improve.

➤ *Mood stabilization.* The ketogenic diet has been shown in studies to be effective in treating mood disorders such as bipolar disorder[20] and schizophrenia.[21]

➤ *Reduction of factors associated with cancer.* A ketogenic diet will cause blood-sugar, insulin, and insulin-like growth factor 1 (IGF-1) levels to drop. Elevated levels of these markers are associated with an increased risk of cancer.[22] Hence, lowering them may reduce your risk of developing cancer.

➤ *Improvement of non-alcoholic fatty liver disease (*NAFLD*).* The ketogenic diet can improve this condition more effectively than a calorie-restricted diet. A study at the University of Texas Southwestern Medical Center found that after two weeks on a carb-restricted diet, there was a 42% reduction in hepatic triglycerides in persons with NAFLD.[23]

As you can see from the list above, the change of lifestyle required to adopt a ketogenic diet is balanced nicely by the benefits it bestows. In the next section, we'll dismantle some of the common myths and misconceptions about ketogenic diets.

Dietary Myth Busting

Let's look at three of the most widespread myths about the supposed dangers of a ketogenic diet. In explaining how each came to be, we

KETOGENIC DIETS AND DIABETES

hope to arm you for the next argument you have with someone who thinks your dietary choices are going to "kill you."

Myth #1: Ketosis is the same as ketoacidosis

One of the most prevalent myths about ketogenic diets is that nutritional ketosis is the same as diabetic ketoacidosis (DKA). In reality, they are two distinctly different conditions.

It's not surprising that medical professionals in particular confuse the two conditions. Medical-school biochemistry textbooks only touch on ketone metabolism briefly. Of the 1,030 pages of the eleventh edition of the *Textbook of Medical Physiology*, one page is devoted to ketone metabolism, a third of a page to ketoacidosis, and four sentences to nutritional ketosis. Incidentally, three of those four sentences are factually incorrect.

Diabetic ketoacidosis has little in common with nutritional ketosis. DKA is a dangerous medical condition caused by a deficiency of insulin often in the setting of illness, typically a serious infection. In contrast, during nutritional ketosis, insulin from either internal or external sources regulates ketone production so that an uncontrolled excess does not occur. If your pancreas is making insulin or if you are healthy and injecting correct amounts of insulin to manage your blood sugar, it's unlikely you would ever experience diabetic ketoacidosis.

Patients with T1DM can develop DKA as a result of an infection, most commonly pneumonia or urinary tract infections, other life stressors, noncompliance with insulin therapy, or as a person's first manifestation of T1DM (previously undiagnosed). The infection or stress causes an increase in hormones that drive up blood sugar. Since the person is ill and may not be eating, they may not realize they need to continue taking proper amounts of insulin.

In a patient with T2DM, DKA can be precipitated by an acute illness such as a heart attack or an infection or, if insulin dependent, by noncompliance with insulin therapy.

Patients with DKA are typically quite ill and require hospitalization with an intravenous insulin infusion along with intravenous fluids to correct dehydration. Although metabolic acidosis causes numerous enzymatic reactions to malfunction, the primary cause of death is not DKA itself but rather the underlying precipitating causes. The physiological factors that precipitate DKA include:

- Uninhibited ketone synthesis (associated with insulin deficiency)
- An inability to utilize all of the ketones produced
- Excess production of glucose-creating hormones (glucagon, cortisol, epinephrine, and growth hormone), which leads to excessive glucose production by the liver.

The symptoms of DKA include the following:

- Polyuria (frequent urination)
- Polydipsia (drinking lots of fluids)
- Thirst and dry mouth
- Nausea and vomiting
- Abdominal pain
- Confusion
- Heavy or labored breathing
- Fruity breath odor
- Fatigue
- Symptoms related to the precipitating condition

Thus, diabetic ketoacidosis is a serious and potentially life-threatening complication of either insulin-requiring T1DM or T2DM caused by an acute illness, previously undiagnosed diabetes, or noncompliance with insulin therapy. In 30%–40% of children and 20% of adults with T1DM, diabetic ketoacidosis is the initial manifestation of the condition. In patients known to have diabetes, precipitating factors for DKA include infections, intercurrent illnesses, psychological stress, and poor compliance with therapy. Urinary tract infection, pneumonia, and other infections account for 30%–50% of cases. Although diabetic ketoacidosis is a life-threatening condition for type 1 diabetics, and

2%–5% die despite treatment, if medical attention is sought early, the great majority recover completely.

The list below shows the levels of ketone concentrations in various body states to help differentiate between ketosis and ketoacidosis. The first four levels constitute varying degrees of nutritional ketosis while the fifth level is the more dangerous ketoacidosis. In addition, the very high ketone levels associated with ketoacidosis will be accompanied by high blood sugars as well.

- Level 1: Negligible levels after a meal: 0.1 mM
- Level 2: Negligible levels after an overnight fast: 0.3 mM
- Level 3: Ketogenic diet (nutritional ketosis): 0.5 to 6.0 mM
- Level 4: Beyond twenty days of fasting: <10.0 mM
- Level 5: Diabetic ketoacidosis: >15.0 mM

Nutritional ketosis is a normal consequence of the keto-adapted individual who is restricting dietary carbohydrates to between 20 to 50 grams/day. Blood-ketone levels during nutritional ketosis are so low (0.5–3.0 mM) that acidosis does not occur. In contrast, DKA blood-ketone levels are commonly much higher, usually above 15 mM. Following a ketogenic diet or living in a state of nutritional ketosis does not increase the probability of developing DKA. The only factors these two conditions have in common are their first four letters—*k-e-t-o*.

Myth #2: Cholesterol and saturated fat are unhealthy

Another myth about the ketogenic diet has to do with fat intake and, in particular, the amount of saturated fat and cholesterol allowed. The general warning you may hear is that eating a diet high in animal fat will clog your arteries with cholesterol and cause heart disease, a story called the lipid-heart hypothesis or the diet-heart hypothesis. There is now plenty of evidence to refute the lipid-heart hypothesis, so let's take a look.

It is a fact that there has never been any scientific study published that links dietary cholesterol and saturated-fat intake to heart disease, even after billions of taxpayer dollars have been spent in an attempt to prove it. In fact, a 2010 meta-analysis by Krauss et al. distinctly destroys any link between heart disease and saturated fat.[24] And a study done by Chris Gardner's team at Stanford University shows that low-carb diets actually improve heart-disease markers over other types of diets.[25] And another specific study done at the University of Connecticut showed that a ketogenic diet favorably affects blood-test results for heart disease in normal-weight men.[26]

Cholesterol Is Good for You

The truth is that cholesterol is a very important substance in the body. We are composed of one hundred trillion cells, each with a cell membrane that forms a barrier so that substances can be selectively transported across the membrane. Cell membranes are composed almost entirely of proteins and lipids, with an approximate composition of 55% protein, 25% phospholipid (a waxy fat), and 13% cholesterol. Almost every cell can create its own cholesterol, that's how vital it is to our health. Cholesterol is also the starting compound for synthesis of many important steroid hormones, such as estrogen, testosterone, progesterone, cortisol, and aldosterone. More importantly, it's an integral part of our brain and is crucial for proper nerve-cell function. Without cholesterol, the human body doesn't do well. People with a disorder called Smith-Lemli-Opitz syndrome have an inborn error in cholesterol synthesis, which results in abnormalities ranging from mild intellectual disability and behavioral problems to physical deformities that are lethal.[27]

USDA Advice on Saturated Fat and Cholesterol

Although the current 2015-2020 recommendations are less stringent, the USDA still recommends that Americans limit dietary cholesterol and saturated fat intake. We are told to limit nutrient-dense foods such as full-fat dairy products and meat and instead consume polyunsaturated oils, a dubious directive at best. This advice is, in part, why so many of us have ended up obese and sick in America. What the USDA doesn't acknowledge is that there is a decided lack of evidence for limiting dietary cholesterol and saturated fat to benefit heart health. A systematic review and meta-analysis published in the *Annals of Internal Medicine* in March 2014 reported this conclusion:

> *Current evidence does not clearly support cardiovascular guidelines that encourage high consumption of polyunsaturated fatty acids and low consumption of total saturated fats.*[28]

Interestingly, it has been known since the 1950s that dietary cholesterol has little, if any, effect on blood cholesterol in humans. The cholesterol you get from your diet is much less than what your liver and other cells will make to maintain your body tissues, because cholesterol is a very important and beneficial substance in the body. Cholesterol acts as a repair substance for cellular damage, so if it is elevated, it may mean that inflammation and tissue damage are present. In other words, cholesterol is just the bandage over an underlying problem of inflammation, which is more likely caused by a high-carbohydrate diet.

There are a great many studies showing that a high-carbohydrate diet and elevated blood sugar and insulin are strongly associated with inflammatory heart disease. For instance, consider the link between HbA1c tests and heart disease. In the EPIC study done at the University of Cambridge in the UK, the researchers looked at the relationship between HbA1c test results and the risk of heart attack. The results were very clear: the higher a person's HbA1c levels (i.e., the higher the average blood sugars and glycation events), the higher the risk of heart attack.[29]

Insulin Resistance, Diabetes and Heart Disease

People with T2DM who are consuming a high-carbohydrate diet commonly have insulin resistance, metabolic syndrome, and undesirable risk markers for heart disease. These markers include elevated total cholesterol and triglycerides, low HDL cholesterol, and elevated small, dense LDL cholesterol, which is a marker of arterial damage and atherosclerosis. This combination of conditions is called dyslipidemia. Insulin resistance and metabolic syndrome are typically part of type 2 diabetes, but, in persons with type 1 diabetes, taking large doses of insulin to compensate for a high-carbohydrate diet and the resulting obesity can result in "double diabetes," the combination of type 1 and type 2 diabetes in the same individual. The following excerpt is from a review article titled "Saturated fat, carbohydrate, and cardiovascular disease" published in the *American Journal of Clinical Nutrition* in 2010:

> *In recent years, there has been increasing concern regarding dietary effects on dyslipidemia, characterized by elevated triglycerides, low concentrations of HDL cholesterol, and increased concentrations of small, dense LDL particles … This metabolic profile is considered to be a major contributor to increased CVD risk in patients with the metabolic syndrome, insulin resistance, and type 2 diabetes. Both increased adiposity and higher carbohydrate intakes have been shown to increase the magnitude of each of the components of atherogenic dyslipidemia. Carbohydrate restriction under weight-stable conditions reduced total:HDL cholesterol, apolipoprotein B, and the mass of small, dense LDL particles … Particularly given the differential effects of dietary saturated fats and carbohydrates on concentrations of larger and smaller LDL particles, respectively, dietary efforts to improve the increasing burden of CVD risk associated with atherogenic dyslipidemia should primarily emphasize the limitation of refined-carbohydrate intakes and a reduction in excess adiposity.*[30]

The typical changes seen when changing from a high-carbohydrate diet to a ketogenic diet include an increase in HDL and a reduction in both small, dense LDL and triglyceride levels. In other words, heart-disease risk markers improve as carbohydrate intake drops. You will see these changes demonstrated in many of the studies presented throughout this book.

Myth #3: Carbs are an essential nutrient for good health

You'll hear this from many registered dietitians because they have been taught that people should eat at least 130 grams of carbohydrates each day to provide glucose to fuel the brain and avoid hypoglycemia. It's an old way of thinking, and it's just not true scientifically.

Essential nutrients are nutrients that your body cannot make, so they have to be obtained on a daily basis from your diet. There are essential proteins and essential fatty acids, but there is no such thing as an essential carbohydrate. When dietary carbohydrates are restricted, the body relies on fatty acids and ketones for fuel. When the body is in ketosis, it has a "glucose sparing" effect. Skeletal muscles burn fatty acids preferentially, which spares glucose for the brain to use. Once a person is keto-adapted, the brain switches to using ketone bodies for 50% to 80% of the fuel it requires; therefore, less glucose is needed. This small amount of glucose needed to fuel the brain during keto-adaptation can be generated internally. Your liver can make all the glucose needed for brain function from glycogen stored in the liver. And, if need be, the body can also make glucose from protein in your food via a process called gluconeogenesis. Hence, carbohydrates are not essential nutrients. Many people, such as the Inuit of Alaska and the Maasai of Africa, live without carbohydrates for long periods of time without any negative effect on health or well-being.

The idea that the brain is completely dependent on glucose is only true if you eat at least 130 grams of carbohydrate per day. A high-carb diet results in your brain becoming "carb-adapted." Blood sugar and insulin will rise on such a diet, and your brain won't have access to ketones to use as an alternate fuel since insulin interferes with ketosis.

We find it puzzling that this 130-gram idea continues to influence dietary advice because the *Dietary Reference Intakes for Energy, Carbohydrate, Fiber, Fat, Fatty Acids, Cholesterol, Protein and Amino Acids*

(Macronutrients) (2005), a reference on which dietitians rely heavily for nutritional guidance, makes the following statement on page 275:

> *The lower limit of dietary carbohydrate compatible with life apparently is zero, provided that adequate amounts of protein and fat are consumed.*[31]

Ketogenic Diets Are Not for Everyone

While we do advocate for ketogenic diets, we also acknowledge that there are health conditions for which they are unsuitable. The contra-indications presented below are based on information from the physician experts in the application of ketogenic diets at Johns Hopkins Hospital and are offered to help you and your physician or health care professional determine if a ketogenic diet is right for you.[32]

Contraindicated Metabolic Conditions

Individuals with these medical conditions should NOT undertake a ketogenic diet.

- Carnitine deficiency (primary)
- Carnitine palmitoyltransferase (CPTI or CPTII) deficiency
- Carnitine translocase deficiency
- Beta-oxidation defects
- Medium-chain acyl dehydrogenase deficiency (MCAD)
- Long-chain acyl dehydrogenase deficiency (LCAD)
- Short-chain acyl dehydrogenase deficiency (SCAD)
- Long-chain 3-hydroxyacyl-CoA deficiency
- Medium-chain 3-hydroxyacyl-CoA deficiency
- Pyruvate carboxylase deficiency
- Porphyria

Note that most of these conditions are identified early in life, although porphyria can develop at any time.

Health Conditions That May Be Incompatible

Talk to your doctor about implementing a ketogenic diet if you have any of the following conditions. Additional health monitoring by your physician may be needed.

- History of pancreatitis
- Active gall bladder disease
- Impaired liver function
- Impaired fat digestion
- Poor nutritional status
- Gastric bypass surgery
- Decreased gastrointestinal motility
- Advanced chronic kidney disease
- Pregnancy and lactation

Part 2

The Ketogenic Diet in Action

3

Getting Ready to Start

For the past forty to fifty years, physicians and dietitians alike have been taught that a high-carbohydrate diet is best, not only for all Americans over the age of two, but also for those with diabetes. When compared to either dietary protein or fat, carbohydrate, especially from refined starch and sugar, requires large amounts of insulin to move the glucose it produces into cells to be metabolized for energy or stored as fat. Thus, of all the macronutrients, carbohydrate places the greatest demand on the pancreatic beta cells. Since carbohydrate is a nonessential macronutrient, and since diabetes is a state of carbohydrate intolerance by virtue of the impaired ability to make, secrete, or remain sensitive to insulin, it makes sense that carbohydrate would be the macronutrient to minimize.

The ketogenic diet may seem extreme to some but not to Hippocrates, who said, "Extreme remedies are very appropriate for extreme diseases."

You might ask, why not just cut out the refined starches and sugar? Well, that would be a great first step and may be all that is necessary for those with mild glucose intolerance. But, as we will see, for most people with diabetes, it may not be enough to lower blood glucose toward normal and protect against the damage of hyperglycemia.

The ketogenic diet that we present in this book emphasizes nutrient-dense, whole foods rich in natural fats and complete proteins, while restricting all foods high in carbohydrates. Once the total carbohydrate load is restricted, blood glucose and insulin requirements come down, stored fat can be accessed and used for fuel, and appetite is controlled by virtue of having restored cellular-fuel utilization. In other words, once your cells' ability to sense energy availability returns to normal, hunger takes care of itself. That's why calorie restriction is not the primary focus of a ketogenic diet.

For those needing to shed excess fat, it is particularly important to mind the appetite signals. Avoid eating out of habit, as an activity, for emotional reasons, or when you are not hungry. In other words, a ketogenic diet won't cure a behavioral or emotional problem, but it will address the abnormal physiology that results from a high-carbohydrate diet.

Goals, Monitoring, and Side Effects

We want you to be successful on the diet, and there are two goals that we think are important to achieve. Before implementing the diet, arrangements should be made to have a health care professional available to monitor your individual progress. Ketogenic diets have very powerful metabolic effects, and medications will most likely need to be reduced or eliminated.

The first goal is to reduce blood sugar and insulin needs and increase ketone levels. Meeting this goal is based on an effective use of protein moderation, carbohydrate restriction, and, if needed, an adjustment in meal size to minimize after-meal blood sugar spikes and associated insulin needs that can derail blood-sugar control. The ketogenic diet is an excellent tool for this purpose because high-fat foods and the right amount of protein are satisfying and have the metabolic effect of reducing hunger.

The second goal is to treat possible side effects associated with starting the diet. Treating side effects includes managing medications and supplements to support dietary goals and adjusting insulin dosing as the diet progresses. We implore you: pay attention to this goal and our warning! This diet is very powerful, and *insulin dosages will typically need to be reduced from the start of the diet.* The same goes for other medications, such as those lowering blood pressure. Please work with your physician to address your medication changes before starting the diet. A 2014 study by Saslow et al. comparing a moderate-carbohydrate diet to a very low-carb diet provided the following algorithm on medication reduction:

> *Metformin was continued for the duration of the study unless the participant or his/her doctor requested it be lowered, at which point the dose was cut in half or discontinued completely. Sulfonylurea doses were reduced in half if the entry HbA1c was <7.5% or discontinued if the participant was on a minimum dose. Sulfonylurea was discontinued if pre-dinner glucose levels went below 110 mg/dL despite prior dose reduction; thiazolidinediones were continued for participants with starting with a HbA1c above 7% and discontinued for those with starting HbA1c below 7%.*[33]

Goal #1: Lower Blood Sugar, Increase Ketones

Your task in adhering to a ketogenic diet is to achieve a state of nutritional ketosis by significantly reducing carbohydrate intake and eating adequate but not excessive amounts of protein. For most people, eating excessive amounts of protein and/or carbohydrate on a daily basis will stop the process of ketogenesis and halt nutritional ketosis. In response, ketone levels in the blood will fall below the level that can be used efficiently by the brain. It may take between one and two weeks of strict compliance to the ketogenic diet for your ketone levels to rise above 0.5 mM. Cheating during this time will have the effect of setting you back to square one. For this reason, it is strongly recommended that you track food and supplement intake in a food log or journal, or use a food-tracking website such as fitday.com, myfitnesspal.com, or cronometer.com.

A simple food log can be kept in a ruled notebook, or you can download a log sheet which is located at the bottom of the About This Site/Resources page of the ketogenic-diet-resource.com website. Record your blood sugars and note the date, meal time, and what you ate. This information will help you determine what foods have negative effects on your blood-sugar control. Ketones can also be measured and recorded as a secondary data point.

Gather Data to Track Progress

Tracking your progress on a ketogenic diet involves three basic activities. First, have baseline laboratory blood tests performed before starting the diet and repeat these tests periodically for comparison. Second, monitor your blood-sugar and ketone levels to determine how your food and supplement choices affect them. Third, make adjustments and troubleshoot.

Keeping a food and supplement log and recording blood-sugar readings on a consistent basis are absolute musts. Checking blood-ketone levels periodically can help ensure that carbohydrate and protein restrictions are adequate. There is just no other way to clearly understand how your food choices affect blood-sugar and ketone values without tracking what and how much you eat and what supplements you take. The other benefit of logging food, supplements, and blood measurements is having this information available to share with your health care professional.

Laboratory Tests

Most health practitioners will want to see the results of your laboratory tests as they work with you on the diet. In addition to the standard diabetes blood tests (HbA1c, fructosamine), a full blood count and complete blood-chemistry panel are helpful to check for kidney and anemia issues. A lipid panel is used to check cholesterol and triglyceride levels, and you may also want to have your iron, magnesium, and vitamin D levels checked. Some practitioners may also want to see a vitamin B$_{12}$ test, and tests for inflammation may also be requested. These may include a high-sensitivity C-reactive protein (hs-CRP) test and other marker tests for oxidative stress, a potent driver of inflammation.

It is again strongly recommended that you find a qualified health care practitioner to monitor your progress.

Tools for Measuring Blood Glucose and Ketone Levels

Accurate blood-sugar and ketone measurements are an important part of managing T2DM with a ketogenic diet. Blood-sugar meters and associated strips are available anywhere diabetic supplies are sold. At this time of publication, there are two blood-sugar meters found to be highly accurate in published studies: the Freestyle Lite and the Freestyle Freedom Lite blood-sugar meters from Abbott Laboratories. Other meters that did well in testing include the AccuCheck Aviva Plus and the AccuCheck Go.[34]

Currently, there are three ways to test for ketones: urine tests, home blood meters, and—the newest method—using a breath-ketone analyzer called Ketonix. Urine-ketone strips are the least expensive option and are available in most pharmacies. They are the best option when beginning a ketogenic diet. In a minority of individuals, urine ketones can decrease due an improvement in the kidney's ability to retain ketones, which results in low or negative urine ketones despite the presence of nutritional ketosis. The Precision Xtra blood-ketone meter by Abbott Laboratories and test strips are more expensive but measure blood beta-hydroxybutyrate levels quite accurately. The Ketonix breath-acetone meter is a one-time expense, making it quite cost effective. Ketonix is also easy and convenient to use. It has not been independently tested against blood or urine measurements, so each individual will need to make one's own correlation between its percentage readout and one's personal therapeutic goals.

We'll talk about measuring blood sugar and ketones in conjunction with a ketogenic diet in greater detail in chapter 8.

Goal #2: Treat Possible Side Effects

Since the ketogenic diet is metabolically powerful, it does come with some potential side effects. As mentioned previously, medication and insulin dosages will most likely have to be reduced immediately.

In addition, while it's unlikely that you or any other person on the diet will experience all of the known side effects, they should be discussed because they can be alarming if you don't know about them. Most of these effects are the result of not getting enough salt and other minerals, and they resolve themselves as the body adapts to the diet. Nevertheless, since they are unpleasant, let's discuss them and review methods for minimizing them.

Possible Side Effect 1: Hypoglycemia (Low Blood Glucose)

If you take insulin or other medications for type 2 diabetes, the dosage will likely need to be decreased as carbohydrate intake is lowered to avoid hypoglycemia (low blood sugar). Particularly for those who take insulin, the mealtime insulin dose will need to be decreased as carbohydrate intake is lowered. As mentioned previously, you should work with your physician to help adjust your medication dosages. Sometimes, basal insulin doses may need to be adjusted as well. Not making these adjustments can result in hypoglycemia, which can be treated by taking one or two glucose tablets (each containing 4 grams of glucose). It may help to reduce dietary carbohydrate levels in stages over several weeks until you can stay at lower carb levels without a reaction. This also applies to those who have experienced reactive hypoglycemia, a condition in which blood sugars dip below normal after a high-carb meal.

Possible Side Effect 2: Hunger and Cravings

Hunger and cravings are normal and are challenges for those new to the diet. Over time, being "in ketosis" and adapting to this shift in metabolism have a pronounced dampening effect on hunger. This is not to say that psychological cravings will also disappear, but the bio-chemical drivers will be greatly reduced. If hunger is still a problem after two to three weeks on the diet, you may be eating too many carbs or too much protein for your individual needs. Review what you're eating from your food log to be sure that your food intake matches your recommended level of macronutrients (see chapter 5).

If you find that you are eating the correct amounts of protein and carbohydrate, recalculate your protein grams for a higher goal weight, and see if the extra protein helps quell hunger. If so, you may be shooting for a goal weight that is too low.

Possible Side Effect 3: Weakness, Dizziness, and Fatigue Due to Dehydration

Fatigue, dizziness, and feelings of weakness or shakiness can be caused by dehydration and mineral loss. Implementing a ketogenic diet usually causes the body to rid itself of excess water and salt due to the effect of lower insulin levels on kidney function. This results in increased urination and loss of electrolytes and minerals such as sodium, potassium, calcium, magnesium in the urine.

It is the loss of these minerals and water that can result in fatigue and other symptoms of dehydration: increased thirst, dry mouth, cramping, weakness, irritability, headache, dizziness, palpitations, sluggishness, and fainting. Replace the minerals and fluids by sipping meat and chicken broth and eating more green leafy vegetables. You can also drink a cup or two of homemade mineral water from the recipe in appendix A or use salt substitutes containing potassium to replace lost salt and potassium. (Warning: if you're taking diuretics or have been advised by your physician to avoid salt, work with your doctor to implement this diet before changing your salt or potassium intake.) You may want to take a mineral supplement:

- To keep potassium levels up, eat more avocado and green leafy vegetables.

- Take magnesium citrate supplements as recommended in appendix A. (If there are kidney issues in your medical history, don't take oral magnesium or potassium supplements without checking with the physician responsible for the care of those conditions.)

- To keep sodium levels up, don't be afraid to add salt to meals. If you experience weakness or a "woozy" or "unfocused" feeling, you can add salt by either by putting one quarter teaspoon of sea salt in a glass of water and drinking it or by having a cup or two of the homemade mineral-water solution in appendix A. Symptoms should improve shortly if a mineral imbalance is the problem.

Possible Side Effect 4: Constipation or Diarrhea

Constipation can be an indication of low magnesium, a side effect of pain drugs, and/or the result of dehydration. Individuals with slow gastrointestinal (GI) motility (due to drugs or disease) should discuss options to address constipation with their physician. There are products recommended for constipation such as Milk of Magnesia, MiraLAX, or Movicol (Polyethylene Glycol 3350) and stool softeners such as Dulcolax. Laxative teas are another option. Examples include Smooth Move® from Traditional Medicinals and Get Regular® from Yogi brand.

Bulky greens such as romaine lettuce and sautéed mixed greens can also ease constipation. Fiber-bulking products such as psyllium husk powder should not be used if you are currently constipated, but can be used after bowel movements return to normal. (See the Dietary Fiber section in chapter 4 for details.) Individuals with ulcerative colitis, Crohn's disease, or bowel obstruction issues should not use psyllium husk. Talk to your doctor about other options, especially if you have any medical conditions.

Although constipation is more common, some people experience diarrhea the first week or two of a ketogenic diet. We believe this may be associated with either a reaction of the gut microbiota to a change in food choices, or excessive magnesium or coconut oil intake. If it is a gut microbiota reaction, it should clear up in a few days.

Possible Side Effect 5: Muscle Cramps

Muscle cramps may result from water and mineral losses that were discussed above. Dosages of diuretic drugs may need to be adjusted as ketogenic diets are naturally diuretic. It's important to discuss this first with your prescribing physician before making changes. For muscle cramps, drink more water and follow the recommendations of Dr. Jeff Volek and Dr. Stephen Phinney in their book *The Art and Science of Low Carbohydrate Living* They recommend taking three slow-release magnesium tablets each day (e.g., Slow-Mag or Mag 64) for twenty days and then continuing to take one tablet a day thereafter to prevent muscle cramps. (Again, individuals with kidney problems should not take oral magnesium or potassium supplements without checking with the physician responsible for treating those conditions.)

Possible Side Effect 6: Ketone Breath

Excess ketones can be expelled from the body via the lungs and in the urine. The main ketone in breath is acetone, which has a distinctive smell. Ketone breath is described as being "fruity" or "metallic." As your body adapts to using the ketones as fuel, less should be expelled in your breath. Although ketone breath may be noticed by significant others, we consider it a good indicator that you've achieved the state of nutritional ketosis. Non-sugar-containing breath mints or mouthwash will effectively disguise the mild odor of acetone.

Possible Side Effect 7: Weight Changes

A ketogenic diet lowers blood glucose, which lowers insulin needs and may eventually lower caloric intake as hunger subsides. If you experience unintended weight loss, eat more calories in the form of natural fats (butter, macadamia nuts, and avocados) on a daily basis until the weight loss stops. If this doesn't help, add an ounce or two of protein to your daily totals.

Possible Side Effect 8: Changes in Blood Pressure

High insulin levels result in greater retention of salt and water. For some people, this excess water storage translates into high blood pressure. Once insulin requirements decrease, the kidneys excrete excess water. Blood pressure should drop as a result. For this reason, a physician should monitor all blood-pressure medication being taken. If you take blood-pressure medication, you may find that you become lightheaded and dizzy after a week on the diet. This is a sign that you may need to reduce your blood-pressure medication dose.

Possible Side Effect 9: Vitamin and Mineral Deficiencies

Vitamin and mineral supplementation is recommended since certain food groups are restricted. A basic multivitamin/multi-mineral supplement that contains the RDA (recommended daily allowance) for all vitamins and minerals is a good start. Pay particular attention that the multivitamin contains the baseline for zinc and selenium. Appendix A lists supplement recommendations.

Possible Side Effect 10: Heart Palpitations or a "Racing" Heart

Some people may experience heart palpitations or a racing heart when starting a ketogenic diet. It's been reported that this is more likely if the person normally has low blood pressure. There are several factors that may be involved in this symptom.

> First, there may be nutrient deficiencies. This is why a multivitamin containing the RDA for selenium and zinc, plus a magnesium supplement, broth, or mineral water are strongly recommended.

> Second, there may be an electrolyte imbalance, or you may be dehydrated. Making some homemade mineral water and drinking

a cup with your morning and evening meal should help if this is the issue. (See Possible Side Effect 3.) In addition, drink plenty of water.

> Third, some people may have "racing" heart reactions to excessive coconut oil or medium chain triglyceride (MCT) oil consumption. If you add these oils to your diet, start with small amounts and increase over time. Don't rely on coconut or MCT oil for your only fat intake. Be sure to include other fats such as butter, ghee, olive oil, and animal fats as well.

> Finally, this symptom may be associated with hypoglycemic reactions as discussed in Possible Side Effect 1.

Possible Side Effect 11: Nausea

Many people are not used to eating the amount of fat allowed on a ketogenic diet. Nausea is common after eating a high-fat meal or a after taking coconut oil or MCT oil. If this happens, try decreasing fat intake and slowly increasing it over time or spreading out your fat intake over smaller meals and snacks.

Final Note on Side Effects and Broth

Many side effects can be managed just by making sure your electrolyte and mineral intake is adequate. Bone and meat broths are a great way to do this. Look for specific bone broth products now available or organic chicken, beef, and vegetable broths without MSG (monosodium glutamate). You can also make your own broth. You can find a multitude of recipes on the Internet with a quick search.

Concerns about Elevated Cholesterol

Many people have trouble on a ketogenic diet plan because they are alarmed about increasing the amount of fat they eat, especially saturated fat. This becomes an issue particularly if their total-cholesterol levels go up and their physicians voice concerns about higher cholesterol levels.

A physician's concern is understandable. The message that eating fat and cholesterol is harmful has been pounded into the collective American psyche for the last forty years. It's also difficult to unlearn the message that high cholesterol is the cause of heart disease. Yes, these messages have been repeated over and over, but they are both untrue. Dr. Ron Rosedale, an expert on ketogenic diets, writes about this myth, and there are several good books on this subject.[35] Nina Teicholz's *The Big Fat Surprise* is one such book. There's also an excellent article titled "Cholesterol: Friend or Foe" written by Dr. Natasha Campbell McBride.[36]

The real culprit of atherosclerosis is chronically elevated blood glucose and insulin, and the associated inflammatory damage to artery walls. This is why diabetics and those with metabolic syndrome suffer from higher rates of heart disease. For most people, following a ketogenic diet over time improves the risk markers for cardiovascular health.

Fifteen Tips for Success

Here are additional tips and techniques for maximizing your success on the diet.

1. You must keep track of what you eat on a per-meal basis, at least at the beginning. Both carbohydrates and proteins must be tracked so as not to go over the daily recommended amount. Keep a spreadsheet, use a web-based food-intake tracker, or keep a written food log or journal. Journaling will help you accurately record food intake, and it can also be used to track mood and physical changes for analysis should there be a need to troubleshoot.

2. Recommended tools include cronometer.com, which offers a ketogenic option, and fitday.com, which offers both a web-based application and an application that can be downloaded to a PC. Myfitnesspal.com is another good choice, and it's free, as are fatsecret.com and the USDA's nutrition database. Finally, the Atkins website also has some nice tools for tracking progress.

3. Get a carbohydrate-counting guidebook or a software application for counting carbohydrates in various foods. Counting carbohydrates is a crucial part of the diet, so it's important to understand how to do this correctly and accurately.

4. Purchase a good-quality digital food scale. It should be accurate to at least one gram. This ensures accurate tracking of food amounts and calories.

5. Go on a carbohydrate sweep. Inspect your kitchen cupboards and refrigerator, removing or separating all high-carbohydrate foods. Restock or rearrange the kitchen so that low-carb, ketogenic foods are readily available. A low-carbohydrate food list is included in the Foods to Eat section in chapter 4.

6. Recognize that a ketogenic diet plan is not a "special diet" that requires special foods. Ketogenic foods are essentially real, whole foods close to their natural state. Avoid low-carbohydrate "convenience foods" such as shakes and bars. They are typically loaded with poor-quality proteins and sugar alcohols that are not healthy and can affect blood-glucose levels.

7. Be prepared to spend more time in the kitchen. This is an important point. A ketogenic diet involves cooking and eating real foods. If you are unable to cook for yourself, check in with your local grocery store and stock up on whole, simple, cooked foods such as roasted chicken and steamed seafood.

8. Think about meal logistics, and learn to plan accordingly. This will help provide a framework to follow, starting with buying the right food at the grocery store. If proper foods have already been selected for dinner, it's easier to avoid making poor selections based on old habits.

9. Replace old habits with new ones. If the normal routine is to visit the nearest coffee shop for a bagel, start making coffee at home and have it with eggs instead.

10. Don't let travel situations put you in a bind. With low-carbohydrate diets increasing in popularity, you can find suitable options almost anywhere in a pinch. Most gas-station convenience stores now carry nuts, cheese, beef jerky, and hard-boiled eggs. See the Travel Tips section in chapter 6 for more information.

11. Stay hydrated. As insulin levels drop, your kidneys will start dumping excess water. At the very least, make sure to drink enough water to replace what is lost. A good general rule is to drink half the number of pounds of your goal body weight in ounces of water each day. Broths without MSG are good choices for hydration because they also provide minerals.

12. Think about social situations that will be encountered. Devise ways to handle temptations to eat the "old" way. For example, a beer with friends usually turns into a dinner of nachos. Think salad and steak instead.

13. Talk with household members. Let them and others know that certain foods are required for adherence to the diet. It is more difficult to follow the diet if someone else in the house has eaten the dinner you had prepared.

14. Monitor your progress. There's nothing like seeing your blood sugar come down—and stay down—to help with motivation.

15. Don't be afraid to eat more fat. Many people have trouble on a ketogenic diet because they just can't get past the idea that eating lots of fat is bad, especially saturated animal fat.

The next chapter will give you some information about the right types of fats and other macronutrients to choose, and what you should and should not eat on a ketogenic diet.

4

Food Facts and What to Eat

Now, let's move onto some general concepts regarding foods you will consume on a ketogenic diet. Remember, there are three main macro-nutrients: fat, protein, and carbohydrate. There are details about various choices within these macronutrient categories that are important for you to know for success, so let's go over them.

About Dietary Fats

Let's talk about fats first because they constitute the majority of the calories you'll consume on the diet. There are several types of fats and oils that have different effects on the body. They fall into three major groups according to their chemical structure. These include saturated fats, monounsaturated fats, and polyunsaturated fats.

- *Saturated fats (SFA)* are solid at room temperature, like lard, butter, and coconut oil. These fats are the most stable chemically and the least inflammatory.

- *Monounsaturated fats (MUFA)* are liquid at room temperature and somewhat stable chemically. These include beef tallow and olive, avocado, macadamia, and hazelnut oils.

- *Polyunsaturated fats (PUFA)* are the least stable of all the fats, since they are prone to rancidity when affected by heat and light. There are two types: omega-6 and omega-3. Omega-6 fats, in particular, tend to be inflammatory to the body. Somewhat less inflammatory are the now-famous omega-3 fats found in fish oil and fatty fish.

Since dietary fats will be a prominent part of your daily meals, they should be chosen with digestive tolerance in mind. Saturated and monounsaturated fats such as butter, macadamia nuts, coconut oil, olive oil, avocado, and egg yolks are tolerated more easily as most people cannot handle eating large amounts of polyunsaturated fats. Examples of omega-6 PUFA include vegetable oils such as soybean, sunflower, safflower, corn, and canola, plus products containing these oils such as mayonnaise and margarine.

Your intake of PUFA from vegetable oils should be minimized. Most nuts and seeds (with the exception of macadamias) are high in omega-6 fatty acids, but they contain many other micronutrients, and their omega-6 content may not be problematic.[37] Omega-3 fats can be found in fatty fish, such as anchovies, sardines, salmon, and tuna, and in grass-fed meats. A good rule of thumb is to emphasize fish and grass-fed meat in your meals, limit nuts to a few ounces each day, and avoid vegetable oils as much as possible.

Natural Fats versus Trans Fats

Contrary to popular rhetoric, natural fats and cholesterol from animal foods and tropical fats from coconut and palm seeds are nourishing and should never have been disparaged or limited in our diets.

In addition to the vegetable-oil fats mentioned above, "bad" fats also include the trans fats, which are man-made products associated with hydrogenating commercial seed oils (e.g., Crisco), and which are included in many processed foods as a substitute for saturated fats. To avoid these fats, avoid foods with the word "hydrogenated" in the ingredients listed on the label. Many studies that originally implicated naturally occurring saturated fats in heart disease looked at them in combination with trans fats, and it was actually the trans fats that had harmful effects on cardiovascular health. When studied in the absence of man-made trans fats, naturally saturated fats do not contribute to heart disease.

Trans fats are finally being phased out of our food supply. This is good news, because trans fats worsen the risk of heart disease by lowering HDL cholesterol and increasing LDL cholesterol along with another heart-disease risk marker called Lp(a) or lipoprotein(a), a subclass of LDL cholesterol. Trans fats are also associated with increased risks for stroke and T2DM. The best way to avoid trans fats is to avoid processed foods altogether.

Coconut Oil and MCTs

Coconut oil is a source of fat on a ketogenic diet that has some special properties. In addition to being a source of long-chain fatty acids, it also contains natural medium-chain triglycerides (MCTs). MCTs have a chemical structure that allows them to bypass normal fatty acid digestion pathways. Instead of being packaged up to travel through the blood, MCTs are passed directly from the intestinal tract to the liver. In addition, MCTs are not stored in fat cells, so they must be burned for energy or converted into ketones by the liver.

The addition of small amounts of coconut oil to your diet will help elevate ketones quickly. However, coconut oil or MCTs can cause diarrhea if over consumed. And, despite the fact that MCTs cannot be stored in fat cells, when consumed in excess, the calories from them can quickly add up and divert other excess calories to be stored in fat cells, contributing to obesity. In other words, if your goal is to lose weight, MCTs will have to be processed before body fat can be burned.

Organic coconut oil is much more available now than it used to be. There are many different brands, and you can buy it online at several Internet sites. Unrefined coconut oil has a strong flavor and odor of coconut. If you prefer a milder flavor, but still wish to experience the benefits of including this MCT-rich oil in your diet, look for "refined" coconut oil.

About Protein

Foods that contain protein are the source of the amino acids needed to create and maintain body proteins. There are nine essential amino acids that our bodies can't create from other nutrients, so they must be obtained from our diet. The daily requirement for protein intake ranges from a minimum amount needed to maintain current function to an optimal amount that allows for muscle growth and repair to support exercise and fitness. For most people on a ketogenic diet, a protein intake should range from 1 to 1.5 grams/kg of goal body weight per day. Consider that range to be a starting point to be adjusted based on your individual needs.

In general, animal proteins are referred to as complete proteins because they have all of the essential and nonessential proteins in the proper ratios that humans need. Vegetables, fruits, and legumes have less protein and more carbohydrate per serving when compared to animal sources. Additionally, plant proteins are often incomplete: they may lack or have smaller amounts of one or more of the essential amino acids.

Protein plays a role in just about every metabolic process in the human body and is required for retaining lean muscle tissue when carbohydrate intake is restricted. It also helps reduce hunger, so make sure you consume protein with each meal. However, don't go overboard. Excessive protein intake necessitates a higher insulin dose than would otherwise be required to control blood sugar. The extra insulin needed to process excessive protein intake also inhibits ketone formation in the liver—not a desired outcome in the treatment of diabetes with a ketogenic diet.

Choosing protein sources that are higher in fat will allow you to have larger servings and still stay within your protein limits. For instance, if you plan to have 28 grams of protein at your meal, a serving of a fatty meat like 80% lean ground beef will be more satisfying than a portion of lean chicken breast because the beef will provide more fat along with the protein. The same goes for a serving of country-style pork ribs instead of shrimp, or a salmon fillet instead of a turkey breast. Go for the dark meat, high-fat choice when you can. The food lists in appendix C provide protein grams and fat grams so you can easily see which protein choices contain more fat.

About Carbohydrates

A quote from the *Principles of Biochemistry by* Albert Lehninger explains in simple terms, one of the reasons why carbohydrates compose 45% to 65% of calories in a standard American diet. Mr. Lehninger wrote:

> *"Carbohydrates per se are not essential in the human diet,*
> *but because carbohydrate-rich foods are abundant and*
> *cheap compared with fats and protein, they naturally form*
> *a major part of the diet in most of the world".*

Dietary carbohydrates include foods containing sugars such as glucose, fructose, lactose, and sucrose. Carbohydrates also include starches, such as those found in potatoes, winter squashes, wheat flour, oats, beans, rice, peas, and similar foods.

Dietary fiber is the indigestible carbohydrate part of plant foods. Its presence can delay glucose absorption and gastric emptying, which blunt blood-sugar responses to the food. Of course, limiting sugar and starch on a ketogenic diet has an even more potent effect on blunting blood-sugar spikes. This is the reason that non-starchy green vegetables—which contain plenty of dietary fiber, vitamins, minerals, potassium, and antioxidants—make up the majority of vegetable choices on a ketogenic diet. Dietary fiber is also fuel for healthy gut bacteria. Gut bacteria consume the fiber and make short-chain fatty acids, which supply an important fuel to cells lining your colon.

Keep in mind that all the carbohydrate our bodies need can be created internally without difficulty. The vast majority of available dietary carbohydrates are not essential to good health. Evolutionary biology teaches us that for 99.9% of human existence, carbohydrates were a small or inconsistent component of our diet.[38] This lesson is especially valuable for those with diabetes.

Remember that diabetes is a state of profound carbohydrate intolerance. It is a simple fact that the more dietary carbohydrate you consume, the more difficult it will be to control your blood sugar.

A study by Boden et al. at Temple University School of Medicine in Philadelphia showed how carbohydrate consumption affects blood-sugar control. Boden's team followed ten obese subjects with T2DM. For the first few weeks, they ate a diet which included 300 grams of carbohydrate each day. During the second phase of the study, the subjects ate only 20 grams of carbohydrate per day. After only two weeks on a low-carbohydrate ketogenic diet containing 20 grams of carbohydrate per day, the blood sugar and insulin responses of the subjects were greatly reduced compared to the levels resulting from the diet containing 300 grams of carbohydrate per day.[39] The authors estimated that if the group had remained on the low-carb diet for eight weeks (the minimum time required for an HbA1c test to reflect the new state of lower blood sugar), the average HbA1c would have decreased from 7.3% to 5.6%.

Consuming refined carbohydrates (e.g., high-fructose corn syrup, fructose, and sucrose) in significant quantities is detrimental to human health. The adverse effects of refined-carbohydrate consumption are even more serious for persons with diabetes. We can't stress this enough, and we strongly encourage people with diabetes to avoid foods containing refined sugars.

Watch Food Labels for Hidden Carbohydrates

Sugars, starches, and sugar alcohols are hidden in all kinds of processed foods and are listed under many different names. Be diligent about reading labels to find hidden carbohydrates. You may recognize some of these common names.

- *Sugars*: glucose, fructose, sucrose, honey, brown sugar, brown rice syrup, beet sugar, coconut sugar, dextrose, molasses, corn sugar, corn syrup, high-fructose corn syrup, fruit-juice concentrate, cane juice, treacle, lactose, galactose, maltose, maltodextrin, hydro-lyzed starch, demerara, turbinado, maple syrup, and agave syrup.

- *Starches*: corn starch, vegetable starch, arrowroot, cassava, ama-ranth, barley, wheat, wheat starch, buckwheat, corn, HVP, HPP, malt, millet, modified food starch, oats, potato, quinoa, rice, sorghum, spelt, teff, tapioca, and triticale.

- *Sugar alcohols*: polydextrose, glycerin, maltitol, mannitol, sor-bitol, xylitol, erythritol, glycerol, isomalt, lactitol, and inositol.

Generally, any chemical name with an *ose* ending is a sugar, and any chemical name ending with an *ol* ending is a sugar alcohol.

Don't rely on food labels to give you accurate carb counts. Food manufacturers naturally have an interest in underreporting carbohy-drate amounts in their products. The USDA nutrition database is a better source for the actual carbohydrate content of foods. Remember to check serving sizes as well. When looking at a large container of yogurt that has 16 grams of carbohydrate per serving, verify the number of servings in the container. If there are two servings, then the total carbohydrate count for that container is 32 grams, not 16 grams.

Dietary Fiber

Dietary fiber is the indigestible carbohydrate part of plant foods. Its presence can delay glucose absorption and gastric emptying, which blunts the blood-sugar response to the food. Dietary fiber is also a food source for your healthy gut bacteria. A byproduct of their consumption of the fiber is a short-chain fatty acid called butyrate. Butyrate has many beneficial effects for the cells lining the wall of your colon—not only is it a source of energy, but butyrate has anti-inflammatory effects.[40]

Ketogenic diets can be low in fiber if you don't eat enough green leafy vegetables. Focus on sources of soluble fiber including non-starchy vegetables, chia seeds, or ground flaxseed. Romaine lettuce can be used to add bulk fiber to the diet, as can spinach or kale.

If you prefer to take fiber separately, try a gentle, soluble fiber such as psyllium husk. Plain psyllium-husk powder is recommended, since products such as Metamucil or its generic equivalents have carb-containing fillers. Keep in mind that psyllium may reduce or delay the absorption of certain medications and is poorly fermented, meaning you'll miss out on feeding your healthy gut bacteria.[41]

As a rule, don't take psyllium supplements at the same time you take other medication or supplements. Take psyllium at least one hour before or two to four hours after taking other medications. Psyllium husk is not recommended for people with ulcerative colitis or adhesions or if you have difficulty swallowing. Also, never take psyllium if you are constipated, as it can cause an intestinal obstruction. In any event, it's best to introduce it slowly.

➤ Begin with one half teaspoon in eight ounces of warm water once a day. Mix it well, and then drink it immediately. (Psyllium thickens rapidly when added to water.)

➤ Over time, increase the quantity until you reach the amount that works for you. Most experts recommend two teaspoons in two large glasses of water per day, as needed.

➤ Always take psyllium with a full glass of water, and drink at least six to eight glasses of water throughout the day to avoid constipation.

Artificial Sweeteners

A recent joint statement from the American Heart Association and American Diabetes Association reviewed five nonnutritive sweeteners that had been evaluated and deemed safe as food additives by the US Food and Drug Administration. The sweeteners reviewed included aspartame, acesulfame-K, neotame, saccharin, and sucralose. The authors of the review did not further investigate the safety of nonnutritive sweeteners as that had already been done by the US Food and Drug Administration. The authors did conclude the following:

At this time, there are insufficient data to determine conclusively whether the use of nonnutritive sweeteners to displace caloric sweeteners in beverages and foods reduces added sugars or carbohydrate intakes, or benefits appetite, energy balance, body weight, or cardiometabolic risk factors.

From the experience of those following a ketogenic diet, eliminating sugar and refined carbohydrates and limiting total carbohydrates will go a long way toward resetting your taste buds so that the real sweetness in natural foods can be enjoyed. You may find that eliminating artificial sweeteners will also help you feel satisfied with the natural sweetness in foods.

Stevia has become popular recently as a natural sweetener, and some food manufacturers have begun adding it to various products. The US Food and Drug Administration has not made a determination as to the "Generally Recognized As Safe" status of stevia, but it has not issued any objection letters for a number of "Generally Recognized As Safe" notifications for stevia sweeteners. Japan and other countries have allowed the use of stevia as a food sweetener for many years and no adverse effects have been reported.

Using small amounts of stevia or sucralose occasionally should have little effect on blood sugar. Blood-sugar testing after use of these sweeteners is advised so you'll be aware of your individual reaction.

Sugar alcohols are another choice of artificial sweetener. Ellen gives the pros and cons of each type of sugar alcohol on her website.[42] Erythritol, in particular, seems to be tolerated more easily than other sugar alcohols. Other types such as maltitol can cause digestive issues when consumed in large amounts, and there are older studies which have shown maltitol and sorbitol to be anti-ketogenic, meaning they interfere with ketosis.

Water and Dehydration

Everyone needs water to replace what the body loses through daily activity. On a ketogenic diet, it is even more important, since the diet has a diuretic effect. Drinking plenty of water also helps to remove metabolic waste from the body and supports many different metabolic functions. It's logical that water is lost when you urinate or sweat, but you may not realize that small amounts of water are lost each time you exhale. You need to replace this lost water to prevent dehydration. We can't emphasize enough how important it is that you drink plenty of water. In addition, your body will need more water if you live in a hot or dry climate, are more physically active, are sick and running a fever, or have diarrhea or are vomiting. Some people may have fluid restrictions because of health problems such as heart or kidney disease. If your health care provider has told you to restrict fluid intake, be sure to follow that advice.

Using Condiments

A majority of condiment foods contain sugar or starchy fillers. For instance, a tablespoon of regular ketchup contains nearly five grams of carbohydrate. In addition, pickles, black-bean sauce, taco sauce, sweet hot sauces, vinegar, salsa, miso, chili peppers, marinades, barbecue sauce, and soy sauce also contain significant amounts of carbohydrate. If you use these foods in more than tiny amounts, you may want to count those extra carb grams. In general, you'll find that condiments that are higher in fat will be lower in carbohydrate. Pesto, mayonnaise, and full-fat dressings that have less than one carb per serving are good choices.

Foods to Eat

The lists below will help you determine which foods to choose for success in achieving lower blood sugars.

Fats and Oils

As we discussed earlier, saturated and monounsaturated fats are healthier overall. We've marked each item below as to whether they are mostly saturated (S), monounsaturated (M), or polyunsaturated (P). Avoid hydrogenated fats, such as margarine and shortening, to minimize trans fat intake. If you use seed or vegetable oils (canola, sunflower, safflower, soybean, flaxseed, and sesame oils) select "cold-pressed" organic brands, refrigerate them and avoid heating them if possible. Some of the more unusual fats listed below can be obtained online.

- Avocado (M) (count carbs)
- Avocado oil (M)
- Almond oil (P, M)
- Beef tallow, preferably from grass-fed cattle (S, M)
- Butter (organic or Kerrygold® brands) (S)
- Chicken or duck fat, organic pastured (S, M)
- Ghee (butter with milk solids removed) (S)
- Lard that is not hydrogenated (S, M)
- Macadamia nuts (M)
- Macadamia oil (M)
- Mayonnaise, no or low sugar (Duke's and Hellmann's brands are low or no sugar) (P)
- Olive oil, organic (M)
- Olives, green and black (M)
- Organic coconut oil, coconut butter, and coconut-cream concentrate (S)
- Organic red palm oil (S)
- Peanut butter (unsweetened) (P, M)
- Nut and seed butters (unsweetened) (P, M)
- Seed and most nut oils (P)
- Dark chocolate (90% cacao) within carb limits (S, M)

Sources of Protein

While not critical to success, choosing wild-caught seafood, organic eggs, and organic or grass-fed animal foods is recommended. Websites such as www.eatwild.com or www.localharvest.org can help with locating local sources of clean, grass-fed meats and poultry.

- *Whole eggs:* these can be prepared in various ways. Try deviled, fried, hard-boiled, omelets, poached, scrambled, and soft-boiled.

- *Meat:* all cuts of beef, pork, lamb, veal, and goat. Look out for added sugar in hams and prepared deli meats. Fattier cuts of meat are better because they contain less protein and more fat.

- *Game meat:* venison, elk, buffalo/bison, and other wild game are fantastic sources of protein, although these meats are usually lower in fat than beef and pork.

- *Organ meats/offal:* organ meats such as liver and heart are extremely nutritious. Roasted marrow bones are an especially fat-rich culinary treat.

- *Poultry:* chicken, turkey, quail, Cornish hen, duck, goose, and pheasant. Free range is better, if it's available. Dark meat is better because of the higher fat content. There is no need to purchase skinless poultry. The skin is rich in fat and protein, and when roasted until crispy, it's delicious!

- *Fish of any kind:* anchovies, calamari, catfish, cod, flounder, halibut, herring, mackerel, mahi-mahi, salmon, sardines, scrod, sole, snapper, trout, and tuna. When buying canned salmon and sardines, favor varieties with the bones and skin. The bones provide minerals, and the skin provides more of the important omega-3 fats. (Exceptions include breaded and fried seafood, which are high in carbohydrates.)

- *Shellfish and seafood:* clams, crab, lobster, scallops, shrimp, squid, mussels, and oysters. (The exception is imitation crab meat; it often contains sugar and gluten.)

- *Bacon and sausage:* check labels and avoid those cured with excessive sugar (maple flavor for example) or containing fillers such as textured vegetable protein (TVP), soy isolate, wheat gluten, or milk protein. Specialty health-food stores carry most brands of sugar-free and filler-free bacon and sausage. Each serving should have no more than one carb.

- *Peanut butter and whole soy products:* tempeh, tofu, and edamame (soybeans) are good sources of protein, but they contain carbohydrates, so track them carefully.

- *Protein powders:* whey, rice, pea, hemp, or other vegetable protein powders can be used occasionally, but read the labels for added sugars. Also, don't rely on them exclusively as a protein source.

- *Nuts and seeds:* macadamias are the highest in fat and lowest in carbohydrate. Pecans, almonds, and walnuts are good choices. Cashews are higher in carbs so track intake carefully to avoid going over your carbohydrate limits.

- *Special note about fried pork rinds:* they have zero carbohydrate and can be used as an occasional snack; however, the protein in them does not contain all of the necessary amino acids. Count the protein grams but limit the amount so as not to displace other complete-protein foods.

Fresh Vegetables

Most non-starchy vegetables are low in carbohydrates and are good choices. You should eat at least 1 to 2 cups of green, leafy vegetables each day to obtain potassium and vitamins C, K, and E. Choose organic vegetables to avoid pesticide residues. If you choose frozen or canned products, read the labels to make sure no sugar is added.

You'll note that winter squashes, potatoes, sweet potatoes and yams, peas, dried beans, corn, and other starchy choices aren't shown in the following list. These vegetables are high in carbohydrate, so it's best to limit or avoid them. In addition, you'll see an asterisk (*) next to the sweeter vegetables, such as onions, shallots, tomatoes, carrots, peppers, and summer squashes. These should be limited, as they are relatively high in carbohydrate, and even small amounts can add up quickly.

This list is by no means exhaustive, so if you have other favorites and they fit your carbohydrate limits, please enjoy them:

- Alfalfa sprouts
- Asparagus
- Avocado
- Bamboo shoots
- Bean sprouts
- Bell peppers*
- Bok choy
- Broccoli
- Brussels sprouts
- Cabbage
- Carrots*
- Cauliflower
- Celery
- Celery root
- Chives
- Cucumbers
- Dandelion greens
- Eggplant
- Fennel
- Garlic
- Green vegetable leaves (beet, collard, turnip, and mustard)
- Green beans*
- Kale
- Kohlrabi
- Leeks
- Lettuces and salad greens (arugula, Boston lettuce, green leaf, chicory, endive, escarole, fennel, mâche, radicchio, romaine, sorrel, watercress)
- Mushrooms
- Olives
- Onions*
- Peppers, hot
- Radishes
- Scallions
- Shallots*
- Snow peas*
- Spaghetti squash
- Spinach
- Sprouts
- Summer squash*
- Swiss chard
- Tomatoes*
- Turnips and turnip greens

Dairy Products

Organic products from grass-fed animals are good choices. Limit cheese to four ounces and cream to one to two tablespoons if you want to stay under 20 grams of carbs per day.

- Full-fat sour cream (check labels for additives and fillers. Look for brands such as Daisy that are pure cream with no added milk or whey—carbohydrates and protein will be low in these products).
- Butter or ghee (organic or Kerrygold brand).
- Organic cream cheese (look for brands without added whey).
- Heavy whipping cream (at least 36% milk-fat content)
- Mascarpone cheese.
- Full-fat Greek yogurt (unsweetened).
- Full-fat cheeses (brie, cheddar, Swiss, colby).

Note that even full-fat dairy products can cause blood-sugar elevations in some people. If you find you are having trouble achieving the blood-sugar reductions you want to see, try reducing dairy products in your diet to see if you get more favorable blood-test results.

Beverages (All Unsweetened)

Beverages should be unsweetened and decaffeinated. Caffeine is restricted because it can increase blood sugar. Below is a list of suggested beverages.

- Water, either plain or with lemon or lime juice in small amounts
- Clear broth, bone broth, or bouillon (no added MSG)
- Coffee
- Black or green tea, or other herbal tea
- Flavored seltzer water
- Almond milk or other nut milks (less than 2 g carb/serving)
- Soy milk (count carbohydrates and protein grams)
- Coconut milk, full-fat canned or the refrigerated carton

Spices

Spices have carbs, so you should count them if you add more than one half of a teaspoon to your meal. Also, read labels on commercial spice mixes, like steak seasoning or Greek seasoning. They usually have added sugar, as do flavored extracts. Some don't, so check labels before you buy. See appendix C for a list of spice carb counts.

Foods to Avoid

The lists below provide guidance on which foods to avoid on a ketogenic diet.

Sugars and Sweetened Foods

Sugar is ever-present in our food supply and not only in candy, soft drinks, and fruit spreads. The only way to avoid it is to eat only fresh, unprocessed foods. If packaged foods are consumed, read the food labels carefully. Avoid any foods that have been sweetened with these ingredients:

- Sugars, such as white sugar (sucrose), brown sugar, cane sugar, powdered sugar, maltose, fructose, glucose, or lactose
- Evaporated cane juice or cane syrup
- Crystalline fructose
- Syrups, such as corn syrup, sorghum, honey, maple syrup, or agave

It makes sense to bypass the obvious sweet foods like cakes, cookies, muffins, and pies, but also look out for foods such as ketchup, soup, bread, and even canned vegetables. Sugar is added to most of these processed canned, frozen, and dried foods.

Starchy Vegetables

Although they do contain fiber, it's best to stay away from these popular starchy foods because of their high carbohydrate content:

- Potatoes, sweet potatoes, yams, and potato products such as hash browns, potato chips, tater tots, and French fries.
- Corn, beets, okra, acorn and butternut squash, yucca, and artichokes.

- Legumes, including most members of the bean and pea families, such as lentils, lima beans, kidney beans, and black-eyed peas.

Processed and Convenience Foods

Processed foods contain chemical preservatives, hidden sugars, and starchy additives. Avoid these types of foods:

- Chips made from potatoes or other starchy vegetables (this includes Terra chips, vegetable chips, crunchy bean pods, and the like).
- Canned soups and stews (most canned products contain hidden starchy thickeners).
- Bagged and boxed processed foods such as Hamburger Helper®, stuffing mixes, puddings, and Jello® gelatin. (Most are high in wheat or sugar and contain added chemicals in the form of preservatives and fillers.)

All Grains and Grain Products

Wheat flour is widely used as a filler in processed foods. Read food labels carefully and avoid or minimize the following:

- Wheat, barley, rye, sorghum, triticale, teff, spelt, rice, vegetable protein, amaranth, buckwheat, millet, quinoa, and corn.
- Products made from grain flours, such as white flour, whole wheat flour, bread flour, oat flour, teff flour, rice flour, soy flour, breads of all kinds, waffles, pancakes, pasta, muffins, cold cereals, hot cereals, bread crumbs, tortillas, crackers, cookies, cakes, pies, pretzels, wraps, and flatbreads.
- Corn products, such as cornbread, tamales, corn chips, grits, polenta, popcorn, stuffing mixes, and cornmeal (corn is in most processed foods as high-fructose corn syrup, as a thickener, or as a preservative).

- Packaged foods that are breaded or that contain breadcrumbs as a filler, such as prepared meatballs, fish sticks, and chicken nuggets or chicken tenders.

Fruit and Fruit Products

While they do have some health benefits, fruits in any form (dried, fresh, or frozen) are high in carbohydrates and fructose. Fructose, even from natural fruit, places a metabolic load on the liver and can drive up blood sugar if eaten in large amounts.

- Bananas, grapes, oranges, peaches, and dried fruit are the highest in carbohydrate. Avoid them, as they will sharply increase blood sugar.
- Berries are the lowest in carbohydrate. If the craving for something sweet becomes overwhelming, try a few strawberries, blueberries, or raspberries, and then test your blood sugar one hour later to see if it significantly increases.

Beverages

These high-carbohydrate beverages should be avoided while on a ketogenic diet:

- Non-diet sodas that often contain large amounts of high-fructose corn syrup
- Sweet alcohol sources such as liquors, sweet drinks, and dessert wines
- Malt beverages and beers
- Juices made from fruits and vegetables that are very high in sugar (several tablespoons of lemon or lime juice are okay)
- Milk (whole, skim, and 2%)
- Sweetened varieties of almond and coconut milk

Tips on Avoiding High-Carb Favorites

Here are some tips on using substitutions to ease cravings for restricted high-carb foods such as bread, crackers and sweets.

➤ Try flavored sparkling water for a fizzy drink. You can add liquid stevia or sucralose for a "soda" experience. Or if you are a fan of sweet-tasting sodas, try the Zevia brand. It's made with stevia. You can also try the Hansen's diet brand, which uses Splenda.

➤ Put one to two tablespoons of heavy cream in a cold glass, and slowly pour in a cold Zevia® root-beer drink for a "root-beer float."

➤ Try adding low-carb syrups to flavor drinks and foods. Da Vinci® and Monin® brands have sugar-free syrups in some great flavors that are excellent when added to a mixture of softened cream cheese, whipped cream, and sour cream to make a dessert. Make sure to order the sugar-free kind as they have the same flavors in their sugar-sweetened form.

➤ If you love bread, you can bake tasty, low-carb substitutes from almond or coconut flour. See the Ketogenic Diet Resource website for some great recipes. Googling "low-carb bread" will provide even more choices. There are many low-carb cracker recipes as well.

➤ If you like cruncy snacks, you can make cheese chips in the micro-wave. Just put a few cubes of colby or cheddar on parchment paper and microwave for about a minute. These are great with homemade guacamole and a little salsa.

➤ Good low-carb mashed potatoes and tasty corn grits can be made by substituting cauliflower in place of the potatoes and corn. Googling should reveal a recipe or two.

➤ White turnips make an excellent potato substitute in hash browns. Simply shred, mix in some shredded cheese and fry in butter. They are great cut into chunks for a beef stew too.

➤ Make "chocolate candy" by melting coconut oil with unsweetened chocolate and ground nuts. Add sucralose and erythritol sweeteners (Truvia®) to taste (the Da Vinci and Monin syrups are also good for this application).

➤ Another idea for candy is to mix softened cream cheese, melted unsweetened chocolate and a sweetener of your choice. Roll spoonfuls into balls, place on a cookie sheet lined with parchment paper and chill until firm. Then dip each chilled ball into melted 85% chocolate and chill again. Keep these in the freezer for a nice treat.

5

Personalizing a Ketogenic Diet

Following a ketogenic diet involves knowing what to eat and how much to eat within the parameters of the diet. The goal of a ketogenic diet plan is to determine how many calories you need to maintain or achieve your ideal body weight, and then figure out the right amount of fat, protein and carbohydrate to eat within that calorie limit. This result should help you get to or maintain your ideal weight while also achieving nutritional ketosis.

In this chapter, we present a step-by-step method we've developed to help your build your own customized ketogenic diet. To begin, let's discuss the three easy rules to follow when implementing the diet.

Start a Ketogenic Diet with Three Rules

Rule 1:

Limit protein intake to what is needed for "repair and maintenance." For most people this will range from 1 to 1.5 grams of protein/kg of goal body weight. Appendix B provides recommended ranges of protein intake based on goal body weight.

Rule 2:

Restrict carbohydrate intake to below 50 grams per day to remain in ketosis, or, if you choose not to enjoy the advantages of ketosis, restrict carbohydrates as much as is tolerable for you. Remember, the more carbohydrates a diabetic consumes, the greater the likelihood of both hyperglycemia and hypoglycemia. This is exactly what we would like to avoid. The carbohydrates you do choose to include in your ketogenic diet should contain lots of nutrients and be lower in energy density. Examples include non-starchy vegetables, nuts, seeds, and low sugar fruits like berries and avocados. Having small amounts of refined carbohydrate junk foods, even if your total falls below 50 grams per day, will not benefit you.

Rule 3:

Dietary-fat intake depends on your weight goals and activity level. Generally, you want to eat enough fat to feel satisfied and maintain a normal weight. If you have excess body fat to shed, you may need to limit dietary-fat intake and calories so that you burn stored body fat instead. Step 4 in the next section will give the details.

Steps to Personalize Your Ketogenic Meals

Below is an overview of the steps that will guide you in implementing a ketogenic diet personalized for your goals and needs.

Step 1: Choose your goal body weight and determine the calories needed to maintain it

Step 2: Find your daily protein intake range

Step 3: Determine your carbohydrate tolerance level

Step 4: Calculate your fat allowance

Step 5: Use your macronutrient amounts to choose foods in the correct proportions

Now that we have an overview of the process, let's walk through each of the five steps using a hypothetical example for our friend Sue Dieter.

Sue Dieter is a thirty-two-year-old female who is five foot six and weighs 150 pounds. Her job is sedentary, but she walks one mile three times a week. She would like to use a ketogenic diet to control her blood sugars, avoid diabetic complications, and take off ten pounds.

Step 1: Choose goal body weight and determine the calories needed to maintain it

Choose your goal weight based on the weight at which you feel best. This may be your current weight or a weight you want to reach. After you decide on a goal weight, use an online calorie calculator (for example, the CI Medical Center has one on their website under "Health Tools"[43]) or use your own experience to determine a daily calorie target. Use your goal body weight in the calculator to factor in your activity levels.

> Sue decides that she feels best at 140 pounds, so she sets that as her goal body weight. She then uses a calorie calculator to figure out a general daily calorie target, and she factors in her activity level to achieve her weight loss goal. Sue looks at the data she gets from the calculator and decides on the calorie goal she will set:
> - Height: 5'6"
> - Goal Body Weight: 140
> - Daily Calorie Needs: 1500

Step 2: Find your daily protein-intake range

As we discussed earlier (Basic Rules for Implementing a Ketogenic Diet), protein intake on a ketogenic diet should range from 1 to 1.5 grams/kg goal body weight per day. The lower end of the range will facilitate weight loss, if needed. However, do not reduce protein intake below 1 gram per kg of goal body weight per day.

If you are consuming 1 gram/kg of goal body weight per day and are still not shedding body fat, then reduce the amount of fat you are eating (which will be discussed in Step 4). In addition, don't go above the top end of your protein range because excess amounts of protein may increase blood sugar. Although there is a table of daily protein recommendations in appendix B, here's how Sue would determine the grams of protein she needs each day.

> Sue set her goal body weight in Step 1 at 140 pounds. She divides 140 pounds by 2.2 to arrive at her goal body weight in kilograms; this equals 63.6 kilograms, which she rounds to 64 kg. At one gram per kilogram of ideal body weight, the now knows her minimum protein intake is 64 grams. She multiplies 64 by 1.5 to get 96, the top end of her protein range. This puts her range at 64 to 96 grams of protein/day.

Step 3: Determine your carbohydrate tolerance level

Your carbohydrate tolerance level can range from 20 to 50 grams per day, with the low end better suited for weight loss. As mentioned, most diabetics would do well to limit carbohydrate intake to below 50 total grams per day to remain in ketosis. If you choose to avoid nutritional ketosis, restrict carbohydrates as much as is tolerable for you.

Although recommendations are to keep carbohydrate intake below 50 grams per day, you can start at 50 to 100 grams per day to allow time to adapt to both the diet and lower blood sugar and insulin. This slower introduction may minimize the likelihood of hypoglycemia and help you adjust your blood-sugar medications. To start slowly, try 5- to 10-gram reductions of daily carb intake on a weekly basis until you reach a low of 20 to 50 carb grams per day. For instance, you might start week one at 100 grams per day. Then during week two, reduce intake to 90 grams per day, and during week three, reduce to 80 grams per day and so on.

> Sue decides to start at 30 total grams of carbs per day. She plans to monitor how she feels and check her blood-glucose response at each meal to assess whether her carb limits are appropriate.

Total Carbs versus Net Carbs

A question we are asked frequently is whether to count total carbohydrates or "net" carbs. In general, many carb counting resources advise that net carbs (grams) = total carbs (grams) minus dietary fiber (grams) minus sugar alcohols (grams).

Dietary fiber is utilized by your gut bacteria to make short-chain fatty acids (acetate, propionate, and butyrate) which are then primarily utilized by your colon cells for energy. Thus, dietary fiber does not raise blood glucose in those with diabetes. In fact, a study published in the *New England Journal of Medicine* showed that subjects with type 2 diabetes experienced a reduction in blood glucose when they consumed 50 grams of dietary fiber per day.[44] In contrast, sugar alcohols (e.g. maltitol, erythritol, glycerol, hydrogenated starch hydrolysates, xylitol) do have absorbable calories and do raise blood glucose and thus should *not* be included in the formula for net carbs.

Hence, we think net carbohydrate should be calculated as follows: *Net carbs (grams) = (grams of total carbs) - (grams of dietary fiber)*. In other words, subtract grams of fiber, but not sugar alcohol carbs, from total carbs when counting.

Step 4: Calculate your fat allowance

Your fat intake is determined by subtracting your protein and carb calories from your total calorie target. Protein and carbohydrates have 4 calories per gram and fat has 9 calories per gram.

> Sue uses the top end of her protein gram range to perform the following simple calculations. Her choice is arbitrary, as she knows she can always reduce protein intake should that become necessary.

> Since protein and carbohydrates both have the same number of calories per gram (4), Sue adds them together. She adds 96 (grams of protein) plus 30 (grams of carbohydrate),

which equals 126 grams, and then multiplies that number by 4 calories: 126 grams times 4 equals 504 calories. So Sue can have about 500 calories of protein and carbohydrate (combined) each day.

Next, Sue subtracts that amount from her daily calorie target of 1500 calories: 1500 minus 504 equals 996 calories.

Sue now knows she can have about 1000 calories of fat each day. She divides 1000 by 9 to figure out how many grams of fat that would be, which works out to about 111 grams of fat each day.

The amount of fat you can eat to maintain ideal weight depends loosely on your energy expenditure and weight status. You need enough fat to get your essential fatty acids and absorb fat-soluble vitamins. Sufficient fat in your diet also helps prevent your metabolism from behaving like it's starving (i.e., slowing down).

Eating an equal or greater amount of fat than you need means your body will use what you eat first, and body fat will either remain the same or increase. Following a ketogenic diet can facilitate fat loss, but it does not guarantee it. A good place to start for reducing fat intake is to cut back on high-fat calorie foods such as nuts, cream, and cheese. If you are not reaching your weight-loss goals, try reducing your daily fat intake by 10 grams (say from 100 to 90 grams) and maintaining this new number for one week. After one week, if needed, reduce the daily fat intake another 10 grams. Continue this weekly reduction process until weight loss begins and then stay at that level.

Correct adjustment of all three dietary macronutrients (carbohydrate, protein, and fat) is necessary for reducing body-fat stores. If you have excess weight to lose, and these steps don't resolve the issue, we recommend you consult with a physician or nutritionist who is knowledgeable in ketogenic diets. A solution is available, but sometimes it takes an expert to sort out the source of the problem. There could be undiagnosed medical problems or medications that need to be addressed that are preventing body-fat loss.

Step 5: Use your macronutrient amounts to choose foods in the correct proportions

Once you have figured out your macronutrient amounts, you can decide how to divide them over the day. We recommend the use of free websites such as myfitnesspal.com or cronometer.com to track your intake and take the aggravation out of staying on target.

Sue now knows she can have the following amounts of macronutrients on a daily basis:
- 64 to 96 grams of protein
- 30 grams of carbohydrate
- 111 grams of fat

Sue divides her target macronutrient amounts and calorie intake by the number of meals she eats. If she eats three meals each day, her targets at each meal might look like this:

Total Daily Calories: 1500 calories divided over three meals each day is about 500 calories per meal

Protein: 64 to 96 grams divided over three meals each day is 21-32 grams of protein at each meal

Carbs: 30 grams divided over three meals each day is 10 grams of carbohydrate per meal

Fat: 111 grams divided over three meals each day is 37 grams of fat at each meal

Using the Food Lists

Food choices are usually a combination of fat, protein, and carbohydrate. We've built some food lists in appendix C that include the amount of each macronutrient for common types of foods. You can also use any food-count book that includes all the macronutrients, or you can use an online food-tracking website such as www.myfitnesspal.com or www.cronometer.com.

If Sue doesn't mind tracking her food intake on paper, she can now go to the food lists in appendix C and pick out the foods she wants to eat that match her daily macronutrient amounts. She can also use a food-counter book or an online food-tracking database to choose her foods.

Making It Easy

Using a tracking website such as myfitnesspal.com makes it easy to select the right amount of foods that fit within your mealtime macronutrient allowances. We highly recommend using this approach as you can readily adjust amounts of each food until you have the right balance of macronutrients. Regardless of how you determine what to eat for each of your meals, it's important that you write down or print out the meals you plan to prepare on a regular basis. This eliminates the need to repeatedly look up or calculate amounts. For every recipe that you have at your fingertips, implementing the diet will become that much easier.

A Few Example Meals for a 150-Pound Person

These meals are designed for a 150-pound person and are in perfect ketogenic ratios. Adjust the amounts for your physical measurements and your custom macronutrient needs.

Eggs and Bacon with Spinach

In 24 grams of butter, sauté about 15 grams of white onion, and cook until soft. Throw in 1 cup of raw spinach, and cook until wilted. Make 2 wells in the onion and spinach mixture, and add a large egg in each well. Cook until eggs are done. Top off with 3 or 4 slices of cooked bacon.

Pork Ribs with Cabbage

Sauté 127 grams of country-style pork rib meat cut into small chunks in 27 grams of butter until almost cooked. Add 85 grams of shredded cabbage, and cook until done.

Beef and Onion with Egg

Sauté 30 grams of onion in 24 grams of butter until the onion is soft. Add 100 grams of 80/20 ground beef, and cook until beef is browned. Add rosemary and thyme to flavor. Finally, add two egg yolks and cook to desired yolk doneness.

Smoked Salmon and Cream Cheese

Combine 120 grams of smoked salmon with 30 grams of cream cheese and 25 grams of white onion. Add dill or other spices to your liking. Wrap spoonfuls of the mixture in green lettuce leaves to make a salmon roll, or pile it on cucumber rounds.

Baked Chicken Thigh with Green Salad

Slice a baked chicken thigh (weighing 150 grams before it was cooked) off the bone with the skin. Serve over a salad of 100 grams of lettuce, 10 grams of sliced onion, and 10 grams of radish; dress with 15 grams of olive oil and 10 grams of red wine vinegar.

Chicken Breast with Onions and Hummus

Sauté 130 grams of sliced, boneless chicken breast and 30 grams of onion in 27 grams of butter until almost cooked. Add 24 grams of classic hummus, and stir to make a nice sauce over the chicken.

Baked Salmon and Broccoli

Lay a 140-gram salmon fillet in a piece of foil, and add 38 grams of butter. Seal foil around salmon and butter, and bake at 350 degrees for about 20 minutes. When the fish flakes in thickest part, it's done. While the salmon bakes, steam 75 grams of broccoli in a double boiler. Serve the broccoli with the baked salmon, ladling melted butter over all.

Tips on Using Your Customized Diet Plan

› Although, as Americans, we are used to using ounce measurements, we think it's much easier to use gram weights when weighing foods, but either will work.

➤ Try not to eat all of your macronutrients at one meal. Eating large amounts of food in one sitting will spike blood sugar and insulin. The goal for blood sugar and insulin is low and steady, so it's important to divide up your total macronutrient intake over several meals throughout the day.

➤ If you like to have smaller and more frequent meals, you may need to divide your carbohydrates up between only a couple of meals and then have no carbohydrates during the other meals. Otherwise it becomes challenging to stick to such small carbohydrate allowances at each meal.

➤ If the foods you like aren't included in the Food Lists, you can use an online food-tracking program or a food reference book that provides carb, protein and fat gram counts for foods.

➤ Mix and match food choices as you wish, as long as you stay within the macronutrient levels for your ideal weight.

➤ Pay attention to tracking your choices correctly. Some food choices will count as a protein and fat or as a combination of protein, fat and carbohydrate. Remember that carbohydrates have to be counted, whether they are consumed as part of a fat or protein food or consumed as a food from the Carbohydrate Foods list.

➤ Think outside the box. Eggs and bacon can be eaten at lunch or dinner, and steak with vegetables makes a great breakfast.

➤ It will probably be easier if you start with using "food units" instead of preparing complex meals that require measuring multiple ingredients. Examples of food units would include eggs, avocados, sausage links, bacon strips, pats of butter, cubes of cheese, shrimp, and hamburger patties.

➤ Choosing fattier protein sources (such as 80/20 ground beef and salmon) over lean meats such as chicken breast and shrimp will make it easier to stay within your protein gram range.

➤ Buy meat in bulk and divide it into smaller portions. For instance, say you can have 135 grams of meat in your meals. Buy 80/20 ground beef in five-pound packages. At home, break it into 135 gram portions, shape each one into a patty, wrap it in plastic wrap, and place the patties in a freezer bag for storage. When you want beef, take one out of the freezer, and you're ready to go.

6

Cooking, Dining Out and Traveling

One of the keys to the successful implementation of a ketogenic diet is choosing and eating fresh food. Cooking skills and making the right choices when dining out and traveling are important, so in this chapter, we will discuss how to prepare and choose the right foods while on a ketogenic diet.

Ketogenic Cooking Techniques

Ketogenic cooking is all about creating meals from fresh, basic ingredients. Each meal should be based on a protein source such as beef, pork, poultry, or seafood, which is cooked or dressed with natural fats such as butter, olive oil, or coconut oil. Low-carbohydrate vegetables and salads with dressings complement the meal. Sauces and dressings are all made of natural fats and added as you like. Sauces and dressings are the key to taking a ketogenic meal from okay to fabulous.

The main challenge in preparing ketogenic meals is to substitute new keto-friendly cooking techniques for traditional cooking methods. For instance, stew and chili recipes usually start with coating the meat in flour. For a ketogenic stew, the flour is eliminated. To thicken stew near the end of the cooking process, some of the cooked vegetables can be pureed with a portion of the liquid and then returned to the pot to make a thicker final product. Another way to thicken stews and sauces is to cook them longer to reduce the water and thicken the remaining liquid.

Beef, pork, poultry, and seafood choices should be prepared using the following methods: roasting, grilling, poaching, baking, sautéing, broiling, and steaming. No flour, breading, or cracker crumbs should be used, as they add carbohydrates. The same methods are good for cooking vegetables too. Be aware that cooking vegetables in water (wet-heat cooking) can destroy the vitamins, so steaming is better. If you are making a stew, at least some of vitamins are recovered because the cooking water becomes part of the final meal.

Useful Kitchen Supplies

A nonstick skillet, a food scale, a high-heat spatula, and parchment paper can be used daily while on a ketogenic diet. You will find that these and other supplies are indispensable for making your life easier:

- Heat-resistant silicone spatulas for scraping all fat from cookware (small ones work great for scooping up salad dressing from the bottom of a bowl)
- Digital food scale with ounce and gram measurements
- Travel cooler and freezer packs for bringing food to work or along on leisure activities
- Small plastic containers with snap-on lids with silicone seals
- Small wire whisks to incorporate oils into a sauce or dressing
- Handheld immersion blender
- Parchment paper for baking
- Nonstick frying pans
- Silicone muffin pans and cookie-sheet liners
- Food processor
- Glass measuring cups in 2-, 4- and 8-cup sizes
- Ceramic quiche pan or deep-dish pie plate
- Single-serving glass bowls with plastic lids
- Krups Egg Cooker (nutritionist Amy Berger of Tuit Nutrition says this is the best thirty dollars you'll ever spend.)

Time-Saving Cooking Tips

If time is short during the week, there are ways to stay on track. For example, you can cook all your food for the coming week on the weekend.

- Roast a chicken, debone it, and make part of it into chicken salad
- Bake a beef or pork shoulder, and slice it for easy snacks
- Make egg salad, tuna salad, and other meat salads; these are easy and fast
- Make stews or beef chili in an electric pressure cooker and freeze them in single-serving containers. The Instant Pot brand is recommended.
- Make homemade hollandaise sauce, pesto, and other fat-based sauces and dressings, and store them in the refrigerator so you can grab a quick spoonful to add to cooked meat
- Find local sources with low-carbohydrate food offerings. A local deli may have chicken salads, baked fish, and other low-carbohydrate choices. Or, look for specialty restaurants that have meat kabobs or chef salads that you can buy on the run.
- Stock the cupboard and refrigerator with easy-to-fix, low-carbohydrate foods: canned tuna and chicken, sardines, or hard-boiled eggs for egg salad. A mixture of mayonnaise and cream cheese makes a great dressing for tuna or chicken salad. Mayonnaise and melted butter mixed together tastes great on egg salad or when spread on hard-boiled eggs.
- If you cook in the evening, make extra servings, and store them for the next meal.
- Prepare vegetable casseroles for a quick side-dish option
- Learn new, more efficient ways to cook. For instance, lay out bacon on a cookie sheet and bake it in the oven. It's easier and less messy than frying it in a skillet.

What if I Hate to Cook?

Grocery stores, Sam's Club, Costco, and other big-box stores offer cooked meats, roasted chickens, boiled eggs, ready-to-eat bacon, packaged deli meats, cheeses, and fresh vegetables. Most grocery-store seafood departments will steam shrimp for you. Canned tuna, chicken, and salmon mixed with mayonnaise and cream cheese and served over cucumbers with avocado make a good lunch choice. Salads with full-fat dressing, avocado, and chopped prepared meats are also a great option.

In addition, you may have a local Whole Foods with a smoked-meat department or a delicatessen that offers a variety of cooked foods. Plain Greek yogurt mixed with your choice of spices and a sweetener is very satisfying as a dessert.

Quick Ketogenic Snack Ideas

- Spread a slice of ham, turkey, or salami with cream cheese or mayonnaise, add a slice of cheese, and roll it up by itself or in a lettuce leaf
- Wrap cooked bacon, tomato chunks, and mayonnaise or cream cheese in a lettuce leaf
- Cut cooked steak, pork, or chicken into small pieces and mix with mayonnaise, sour cream, cream cheese, or avocado
- Deviled eggs, or hard-boiled eggs sliced and spread with mayonnaise or sour cream
- Thin slices of smoked salmon spread with cream cheese mixed with dill and lemon juice
- Smoked salmon mixed with scrambled eggs and topped with softened cream cheese
- Baked chicken wings (no breading) and blue-cheese dip
- Crab meat mixed with cream cheese and lemon juice on cucumber slices
- Shrimp with minced onion, mayonnaise, and dried dill on cucumber slices

- Beef jerky cured without sugar
- Antipasto made from peppers, olives, prosciutto or salami, and cheese cubes
- Tuna mixed with mayonnaise and cream cheese and piled on cucumber rounds
- Olives stuffed with feta cheese
- Roasted or raw nuts
- Dill pickles with cheddar cheese
- Pork rinds dipped in a mixture of full-fat sour cream and low-carbohydrate salsa
- Pork rinds dipped in ranch dressing or pesto sauce
- Jicama, radishes, or turnip sticks with full-fat sour-cream dip or ranch dressing
- Celery stuffed with a cream cheese/blue-cheese mixture
- Celery stuffed with cream cheese mixed with curry or any other spice you like
- Celery stuffed with almond butter
- Macadamia nuts fried in butter and sprinkled with cinnamon
- Pecans with thin slices of blue cheese
- Chunks of avocado and tomatoes mixed with mayonnaise
- Steamed or boiled shrimp with dill mayonnaise
- String cheese and pepperoni slices
- Cucumber and tomato chunks with feta cheese and balsamic vinegar
- Sliced radishes spread with cream cheese and sprinkled with chives or spices
- Shrimp mixed with a low-carb Thai green-chili sauce and sprinkled with cilantro
- Crispy cooked bacon mixed with blue cheese and sour cream, then add spices to taste (this makes a good dip for raw broccoli and cauliflower or leftover cooked chicken)
- Two ounces of cream cheese mixed with two tablespoons heavy cream, a little grated 90% chocolate and sweetener

- Low-carb, sugar-free popsicles
- Greek yogurt mixed with cardamom, ginger, cinnamon, and sweetener
- Two ounces of goat cheese mixed with with a few blueberries and artificial sweetener

Recipe Resources

The following recipe sites are useful as a guide. Typing "low-carbohydrate recipes" into Google will provide more sites with recipes to peruse as well.

- www.ketogenic-diet-resource.com/low-carb-recipes.html
- www.charliefoundation.org/
- www.atkins.com/recipes.aspx
- www.genaw.com/lowcarb/
- www.yourlighterside.com
- www.comfybelly.com/2012/06/baking-with-coconut-flour-2/ (for a page on baking with coconut flour)
- www.comfybelly.com/2009/01/baking-with-almond-flour/ (for a post on cooking with almond flour)
- www.ibreatheimhungry.com
- www.authoritynutrition.com/101-healthy-low-carb-recipes/
- www.alldayidreamaboutfood.com/
- www.healthyindulgences.net/
- www. amongfriends.us/
- www.uplateanyway.com/keto/

Low-Carbohydrate Cookbooks

These books provide more ideas for meal planning and include techniques for preparing foods. Not all of the recipes are specifically ketogenic, but they should help in generating ideas for variety in your meals.

- *The Ketogenic Kitchen* by Patricia Daly and Dominic Kemp
- *Low-Carb Gourmet* by Karen Barnaby

- *Fat Fast Cookbook* by Dana Carpender
- *500 Low-Carb Recipes* by Dana Carpender. This goes in and out of print.
- *200 Low-Carb, High-Fat Recipes: Easy Recipes to Jumpstart Your Low-Carb Weight Loss* by Dana Carpender
- *300 15-Minute Low-Carb Recipes* by Dana Carpender
- *Eating Stella Style* by George Stella
- *George Stella's Livin' Low Carb* by George Stella and Cory Williamson
- *New Atkins for a New You Cookbook* by Colette Heimowitz
- *Paleo Cooking* by Elana Amsterdam
- *Low Carbing Among Friends (all volumes)* by Jennifer Eloff
- *Nourished: A Cookbook for Health, Weight Loss, and Metabolic Balance* by Judy Barnes Baker, Jacqueline Eberstein, RN, and Richard Feinman, PhD
- *Carb Wars: Sugar is the New Fat* by Judy Barnes Baker
- *The Low-Carb Comfort Food Cookbook Paperback* by Ursula Solom, Mary Dan Eades, and Michael R Eades
- *Extreme Lo-Carb Cuisine: 250 Recipes With Virtually No Carbohydrates* by Sharron Long
- *Muffins to Slim By: Fast Low-Carb, Gluten-Free Bread & Muffin Recipes to Mix and Microwave in a Mug (Volume 1)* by Em Elless
- *The Low Carb High Fat Cookbook: 100 Recipes to Lose Weight and Feel Great* by Sten Sture Skaldeman
- *Fat: An Appreciation of a Misunderstood Ingredient, with Recipes* by Jennifer McLagan
- *The Keto Cookbook* by Dawn Martenz. There is a Kindle and paperback version. The paperback version is better, as the Kindle version is not formatted in a way that is easy to use.

In addition, most whole-food recipes from your favorite cookbook can be adapted to a low-carb, ketogenic version.

Dining Out on a Ketogenic Diet

Many people want to know if they can eat at restaurants while on a ketogenic diet. The short answer is yes! You can enjoy dining out while on a ketogenic diet, provided you're careful about what you order. Being on this diet should not prevent you from enjoying a nice meal with friends and family. Don't be shy about customizing your order and asking for substitutions when necessary. As people become more health conscious and food allergies become more common, waitstaff are not put off by special requests. Here is a guide to selecting appropriate foods that will allow you to continue getting the benefits of your unique diet.

General Tips

Your best bet for staying on plan is to choose simply prepared dishes. Foods which have been grilled, baked, or roasted meats, poultry, seafood, non-starchy vegetables, or salads are good choices. Low fat salad dressings usually contain sugar, so select either full fat kinds or oil and vinegar. In addition, avoid all pasta, rice, bread, potatoes, corn, beans, soda, and desserts (including fruit). You should also avoid sauces and soups which are usually flavored and thickened with sugar, flour, or cornstarch.

Another good strategy is to prepare before you go! Most restaurants have their menus posted online. Look in advance to see what will be suitable for you so you'll have an easier time ordering. If you're dining with friends and the restaurant of choice isn't conducive to a low-carb meal, simply suggest a change of location.

Tips for Specific Cuisines

> ▸ *Mexican*: Fajitas are a great choice; decline the chips and tortillas, and ask for extra vegetables instead of beans and/or rice. Fajita fillings are just grilled meat and vegetables, and you can enjoy

sour cream and small amounts of cheese, guacamole, and pico de gallo as condiments. Be sure there's no corn in the pico de gallo. (At Chipotle and Qdoba, you can get meat, lettuce, and vegetables in a bowl rather than in a tortilla.)

> *Middle Eastern/Greek*: Choose kebabs or other grilled-meat dishes. Ask for extra vegetables or meat instead of rice or pita bread. Avoid hummus, stuffed grape leaves (they usually contain rice), anything else with beans, and high-starch foods such as potatoes.

> *Chinese/Japanese*: Ask for your dishes to be prepared steamed or with no sauce. (Sauces typically contain sugar and corn starch.) Use soy sauce or hot mustard as condiments. Great choices for Chinese takeout are steamed chicken or shrimp with mixed vegetables. Some restaurants also offer grilled chicken/beef on skewers. Avoid rice, noodles, wontons, dumplings, deep-fried foods, and tempura (due to the breading). Sashimi and sushi are tasty; just avoid the rice.

> *Italian*: Pasta is obviously not permitted, but most Italian restaurants have many other options that are suitable for a very low-carbohydrate diet. Choose salads, steaks, chicken, pork, or seafood with vegetables. Avoid bread and breadsticks, and ask for no croutons on your salad. Ask for extra non-starchy green leafy vegetables as side dishes instead of pasta or potatoes. Antipasto (an olive, meat, and cheese platter) is also a good option.

> *Diner/American bistro*: These restaurants usually have a very diverse menu, and finding suitable options will be easy. Just use the same logic as for anywhere else: no grain or other starchy carbohydrates and no sweets for dessert. Fantastic choices are Cobb, chef, or Caesar salads (no croutons) with full-fat dressing. Perfectly fine choices are hamburgers or sandwiches without the bun or bread. Always ask for non-starchy vegetables (like greens) instead of fries or other potato sides. You can often substitute a simple house salad for a starchy side dish. Other good selections include any type of roasted meat, chicken, or fish or a platter of egg or tuna salad on a bed of lettuce.

➤ *Breakfast*: Stick with eggs, bacon, ham, and sausage. Avoid pancakes, waffles, potatoes, toast, bagels, muffins, fruit, juice, and jam or jelly. Western omelets are a great option (eggs, ham, onion, peppers), as are any type of omelet that contains eggs, meat, cheese, and/or low-starch veggies (peppers, spinach, mushrooms, onions, zucchini). Other types of eggs are great, too: poached, scrambled, over easy, or hard-boiled. Avoid bottled ketchup that contains high-fructose corn syrup. Use mustard, mayonnaise, or hot sauce as condiments.

➤ *Salads*: Customize your salad as necessary—no dried cranberries, fruit, croutons, or crunchy noodles. Stick with lettuce, spinach, and other greens. Suitable additions are chopped hard-boiled egg, bacon, cheese, avocado, ham, turkey, chicken, steak, salmon, olives, cucumbers, sliced peppers, radishes, and other non-starchy vegetables. Use oil and vinegar or a high-fat dressing like ranch or blue cheese. Avoid thousand island, French, honey mustard, raspberry vinaigrette, and other sweetened dressings. (Besides olive oil, you can use avocado or macadamia oil to make delicious homemade vinaigrettes.)

➤ *Chain restaurants*: You can find suitable choices at chain restaurants like Applebee's, Chili's, Olive Garden, and Outback Steakhouse. Just ask for the appropriate substitutions. For example, ask for double broccoli instead of a potato, and avoid the bread they bring as an appetizer.

Beware of Hidden Dining Pitfalls

Restaurant staff use many different techniques to prepare and present food. Sugar is often added to enhance flavors. Don't be shy about asking your server for details on how foods are prepared. For example, some restaurants add flour or pancake batter to their eggs to make omelets fluffier. Ask if this is the case, and, if so, ask if they'll prepare your eggs without that. (Another way around this is to stick with eggs that are hard-boiled, poached, over easy, or sunny-side up.)

If there is a sauce with ingredients that you're not sure of, ask the server to tell you what's in it. Many sauces contain sugar, corn syrup, corn starch, and/or flour. It's best to stay with simply prepared dishes to avoid this.

Be careful with condiments. Ketchup is generally loaded with high-fructose corn syrup, and many salad dressings are high in sugar and corn syrup. Your best bets for condiments (if you need them at all) are the ones listed here:

- Mustard (any kind except honey mustard)
- Mayonnaise
- Hot sauce
- Melted butter
- Olive oil
- Macadamia oil
- Vinegar (red wine, apple cider, white)

Full-fat, low-carbohydrate salad dressings are also permitted. Look at labels in supermarkets to determine which types are best. The carbohydrate count in a 2-tablespoon serving should be 2 grams or less.

The next section offers some tips on staying on plan while traveling by car and airplane and how to handle conferences and social events.

Travel Tips

With thanks to Miriam Kalamian of Dietarytherapies.com, the tips below will help you stay on track if you have to travel. We've tried to cover various travel situations, including how to avoid the high-carb options offered at conferences.

Automobile

- Pack a cooler with small plastic containers of your favorite meals. You are less likely to stray from your plan if you have familiar foods at hand.

- Bring water, and stay well hydrated!
- Carry small packages of nuts and individually wrapped cheese sticks. This is also a good idea when flying.

Air Travel

- TSA may allow food and liquids for consumption during your flight if you notify them that you have diabetes. Call first to be sure; rules change over time.
- Choose salads with protein (chicken, boiled egg, deli ham, sliced cheese) at the airport. Choose salad dressings with the least amount of carbohydrate per serving. Look for mayonnaise packets to use with the protein. You can also eat chilled butter pats.
- Pack protein powder in sealable plastic sandwich bags and bring a plastic shake-maker bottle. In a pinch, you can make a shake with water.
- If you're checking a bag, you can bring your favorite (unopened) salad dressing and a jar of olives. Triple bag this in plastic and add a note explaining what it is (TSA may want to know). Bring clean plastic bags to bottle leftovers for the return trip.

Conferences

Standard meals offered at conferences are a mine field! Ask about food options when you register.

- If you are attending a conference which spans several days, visit the closest local grocery store once you arrive and buy some non-perishable foods such as jerky or nuts, or bring them from home. If you have access to a refrigerator in your hotel room, buy lunch meat and cheese slices to have on hand.
- Breakfast: Stick to scrambled or boiled eggs with bacon, sausage, or cheese. Eat chilled butter pats for extra fat. Ask for half-and-half or heavy cream instead of milk or creamer.
- Lunch: Choose deli meats, tuna, or chicken salad. Scrap the bread

and double the salad veggies (minus carrots). Look for olive oil and vinegar (avoid balsamic).

- Dinner: Choose simple, whole meats, grilled veggies, no sauces, no breading. Add olive oil and/or butter. Make sure you get all the oils from the bottom of the plate or bowl.
- Snack: Macadamia nuts are perfect! You may also want to take along individually wrapped cheddar cheese pieces.

Social Events

- Bring your own meal or eat before you arrive. It's difficult to fight off the "Please, just have one bite" or "But I made this just for you" comments if you're hungry or don't have an alternative.

Part 3

Managing Blood Sugar and Insulin

7

Type 2 Diabetes Mellitus and Insulin Resistance

Type 2 diabetes mellitus (T2DM) is a disorder with at least four contributing causes, including genetic predisposition, intrauterine environment, dietary patterns, and physical activity. Research has shown that insulin resistance occurs years before the development of glucose intolerance, prediabetes, and T2DM. Although insulin resistance is not completely understood, it is a condition in which the body's tissues become insensitive or numb to elevated insulin levels—initially as episodic incidents and, later, as constantly elevated insulin levels resulting from a diet high in refined carbohydrates and sugars. Excess calorie intake may play a role in this scenario as well.

As insulin resistance worsens, the beta cells in the pancreas have to work harder and harder to make enough insulin to lower the blood sugar. Eventually, they can no longer keep pace, and this results in elevated blood sugars—initially, after meals and, later, fasting blood sugars become elevated as well. This is when prediabetes is diagnosed, many years after insulin resistance and hyperinsulinemia have been doing damage to your body. This is, as we have mentioned earlier, why many people develop atherosclerotic heart and vascular disease, stroke, high triglycerides, high blood pressure, metabolic syndrome, cancer, and numerous other conditions prior to the development of T2DM.

This, however, is the reason that these conditions are associated with each other: they all have the common condition of insulin resistance.

Insulin Resistance: An Important Treatment Target

Insulin resistance is defined as a lack of cellular response to insulin signaling, which leads to a compensatory increase in insulin secretion from the pancreas (hyperinsulinemia) and, eventually, in blood glucose when the pancreatic beta cells can no longer keep pace. It is the chief hallmark of metabolic syndrome, prediabetes and T2DM.

There is lack of complete agreement among medical scientists as to the cause of insulin resistance. Some believe it is related to dietary caloric excess and obesity, but normal-weight individuals can have insulin resistance as well.

Others believe it is related to physical inactivity. It is certainly true that regular physical activity improves insulin sensitivity and has numerous health benefits; however, there is little evidence that insulin resistance is caused by physical inactivity. As an example, Dr. Peter Attia, author of The Eating Academy blog, developed insulin resistance and metabolic syndrome even though he exercised four hours each day.

We are of the opinion that carbohydrate consumption in excess of one's tolerance is the most likely cause of insulin resistance, glucose intolerance, prediabetes, metabolic syndrome, and T2DM. This is why carbohydrate restriction with a ketogenic diet alone can reverse these conditions if initiated early in the course of the condition. Exercise alone will not reverse these conditions but should be added to carbohydrate restriction once health has improved. Dr. Attia was able to reverse his metabolic syndrome by adding a ketogenic diet to his exercise routine.[45]

If your blood glucose, HbA1c, or oral glucose-tolerance test (OGTT) results are elevated even slightly, or meet the criteria for prediabetes or diabetes, take that as a sign to change your eating habits and set a goal to normalize your blood glucose. Making changes now may help you avoid permanent damage to your metabolic health later.

Metabolic Syndrome (MetS)

Dr. Gerald Reaven first described Syndrome X (now known as metabolic syndrome or insulin-resistance syndrome) in 1988. He defined it as the presence of glucose intolerance, increased triglycerides, decreased HDL cholesterol, increased waist circumference and hypertension (high blood pressure), and he was able to document that these signs were associated with insulin resistance and compensatory hyperinsulinemia. He thought insulin resistance was the most important feature of Syndrome X and that it was involved as a cause of T2DM, hypertension, and coronary artery disease.

The name Syndrome X was later changed to metabolic syndrome to avoid confusion with cardiac syndrome X. It has also been called insulin-resistance syndrome as well as other similar names. A paper by Grundy et al. explains the components of metabolic syndrome in more detail. Pertinent markers include abdominal obesity, elevated triglycerides, suboptimal HDL cholesterol, elevated blood pressure and elevated blood glucose.[46] The presence of any three of these five criteria defines metabolic syndrome. Why is this important to know? If you have any of the components of metabolic syndrome, and especially if you have any three of the five criteria, you have a significantly increased risk of developing diabetes, cardiovascular disease (CVD), having a heart attack or stroke, and dying at a younger age.

MetS: Are Normal Blood-Sugar Guidelines Too High?

A national study published in 2010 determined that 34% of the US population had metabolic syndrome.[47] This is a staggering figure given metabolic syndrome is linked to an increased risk for T2DM, CVD and a host of other conditions including polycystic ovary syndrome (PCOS), fatty liver disease, cholesterol gallstones, asthma, sleep disturbances like sleep apnea, and some forms of cancer. In addition, there are many studies that show that those with a fasting plasma glucose greater than 85 mg/dL or an HbA1c greater than 4.7% are at increased risk of developing T2DM and coronary heart disease in the future.[48, 49, 50]

This evidence is particularly troubling because it supports the contention that the upper cutoff of the current medical definition of "normal" fasting plasma glucose (<100 mg/dL) is too high.

Detecting metabolic syndrome in patients should be a routine part of a medical evaluation and reversing each of the components of metabolic syndrome is important for anyone who values their health and wishes to avoid future development of CVD, diabetes, and other chronic diseases. Fortunately, the ketogenic diet is very effective in reversing all of the components of metabolic syndrome and its associated chronic diseases.

Prediabetes and ADA Recommendations

In their diabetes basics guide, the American Diabetes Association (ADA) defines prediabetes as an elevation of fasting blood glucose above normal (i.e. >100 mg/dL) but less than the criteria for diabetes (i.e. <126 mg/dL).[51] Prediabetes also increases the likelihood of developing future CVD and diabetes. The table below lists blood-glucose and HbA1c values that define normal, prediabetes, and diabetes that are currently accepted by the American Diabetes Association.[52] The American College of Clinical Endocrinologists (AACE) also endorses similar recommendations.[53]

Diagnostic Criteria Based on Fasting Blood Glucose		
	ADA	AACE
Normal blood sugar range:	<100 mg/dL	<100 mg/dL
Prediabetic range:	101–126 mg/dL	101–126 mg /dL
Diabetic range:	≥126 mg/dL (7.0 mmol/L)	≥126 mg/dL (7.0 mmol/L)

Blood-sugar levels peak at one to two hours after a carbohydrate meal in both normal and diabetic individuals. Using carbohydrate restriction can control the postprandial (after meal) increase in blood glucose and insulin secretion. It can also reduce both blood-sugar and insulin levels, thereby improving HbA1c test results. Ultimately, adopting a ketogenic or carbohydrate-restricted diet can improve all diabetic health markers, including fasting, postprandial, and between-meal blood sugars, and HbA1c. The long-term result is a reduction in glycation damage, which reduces the likelihood of future diabetic complications. Hence, we think aiming for a blood-glucose target as close to the nondiabetic range as can be accomplished safely is a goal worth pursuing for long-term positive health benefits. A ketogenic diet can make this goal easier to achieve.

We find it interesting that the current 2017 American Diabetes Association guidelines for glycemic control in people with diabetes are as follows:

- A reasonable A1C goal for many nonpregnant adults is <7% (53 mmol/mol).

- Providers might reasonably suggest more stringent A1C goals (such as <6.5% [48 mmol/mol]) for selected individual patients if this can be achieved without significant hypoglycemia or other adverse effects of treatment (i.e., polypharmacy). Appropriate patients might include those with short duration of diabetes, type 2 diabetes treated with lifestyle or metformin only, long life expectancy, or no significant cardiovascular disease.

- Less stringent A1C goals (such as <8% [64 mmol/mol]) may be appropriate for patients with a history of severe hypoglycemia, limited life expectancy, advanced microvascular or macrovascular complications, extensive comorbid conditions, or long-standing diabetes in whom the goal is difficult to achieve despite diabetes self-management education, appropriate glucose monitoring, and effective doses of multiple glucose-lowering agents includ-ing insulin.[54]

Why don't the American Diabetes Association and the American College of Clinical Endocrinologists endorse normal blood-glucose values? We think it's because trying to achieve that level of blood glucose control while consuming their recommended high-carb diet and taking insulin and/or oral hypoglycemic medications *is not possible* without numerous and potentially dangerous hypoglycemic episodes. These organizations don't want to recommend a treatment plan that would cause life-threatening hypoglycemia for which they may be culpable, even if it means that patients suffer long-term complications of diabetes from chronically elevated blood sugars.

Although these recommendations are understandable in the context of a diet containing the currently recommended intake of 45–60 grams of carbohydrate in each meal, we believe a ketogenic diet could offer those with diabetes an effective tool for better control of both hyperglycemia and hypoglycemia and a significant reduction in the long-term diabetic complications associated with glycation damage.

8

Blood-Sugar Management for T2DM

In this chapter, we'll discuss the skills and tools needed for managing blood sugar and the importance of accurate blood-sugar monitoring and testing in the prevention of long-term diabetic complications. We'll also present symptoms of and treatment for hypoglycemia and hyperglycemia, and we'll discuss the benefits and drawbacks of HbA1c and fructosamine testing.

Blood-Glucose Management Skills

In order to improve blood-sugar control, patients need to be motivated to make beneficial lifestyle and disease management changes. Managing diabetes is a twenty-four-hour-a-day activity. You may not need to spend more than several minutes each day doing it, but everything you eat and each physical activity in which you partake must be considered in light of its effect on your blood sugar. Under the direction of their physicians, patients must be able to implement and maintain changes by themselves or with the assistance of a close family member or friend. Factors to consider include vision, manual dexterity, mental comprehension, discipline, and compliance. For example, if the patient is taking insulin and has limited sight, being physically able to inject the correct amount and type of insulin can be challenging. Mistakes in administering the amount or type of insulin can have serious adverse outcomes such as hypoglycemia. This is just one of numerous barriers to achieving improved blood glucose. There are many other abilities needed to manage diabetes successfully:

- Measure blood glucose and ketones
- Take insulin and/or medications accurately and consistently
- Select appropriate foods for a ketogenic diet
- Follow diet guidelines accurately and consistently
- Negotiate eating outside the home in restaurants, at the homes of others, and during travel
- Have health monitored by your physician

We suspect that most people reading this book are highly motivated individuals who will follow the steps necessary to monitor and control their blood sugar. It is these individuals who can most likely achieve their target blood glucose without adverse events. Imagine if one in four of the 382 million people with diabetes could achieve much improved or normal blood glucose, there would be a tremendous reduction in suffering, disease burden, and cost of care. That would make for 96 million people who would effectively have their complications of diabetes either arrested or reversed!

Using Blood-Glucose Meters

Achieving optimal blood-sugar control requires frequent blood-glucose measurements. Therefore, having one or more accurate blood-glucose meters is important. Carrying a meter at all times is recommended, especially if you are newly diagnosed or are making changes in insulin type or dose, in diet or in exercise. Keeping an extra meter at work, at bedside, or in the car (unless temperatures are extreme) will serve as a backup if you forget to take your meter with you. Note that the cost of a meter is relatively small compared with the cost of strips used in the meters to measure blood glucose.

Any readings that seem out of the ordinary should be rechecked after washing your hands to remove traces of food or glucose or be rechecked with the use of a different meter. Sometimes, an unusual reading is caused by a defective glucose meter strip, but that is usually indicated by an error code. In that case, simply use a new test strip.

Some meters are more accurate than others. It is a good idea to periodically research the accuracy of currently marketed blood-glucose meters. Searching www.pubmed.gov, using the keywords "blood-glucose meter accuracy" should yield some helpful information.

Real-Time Continuous Glucose Monitors

A real-time continuous glucose monitor (rt-CGM) is a device with a tiny glucose sensor inserted under the skin to measure glucose levels in tissue fluid instead of blood. The device provides a glucose reading on a portable display every five minutes. Some monitors can signal an alarm for preset low or high glucose readings, and others can also communicate with an insulin pump and send a low-blood-glucose signal to suspend insulin pump infusion.

The rt-CGM must be calibrated with a home blood-glucose monitor result at least twice a day. It is not designed to replace home blood-glucose monitoring. Tissue-fluid readings can give a close estimate of blood glucose, but the rt-CGM can be less accurate and has been shown to lag when compared to blood-glucose readings. Nevertheless, it can provide valuable information, including the direction that blood-glucose levels are heading and, thus, provide early notification of oncoming lows and highs. In addition, it can provide information on how food, physical activity, stress, sleep, medication, and illness affect your diabetes, as well as provide estimates of glucose readings at crucial points during the day. Before making any adjustment in insulin or medications, an rt-CGM glucose reading should be confirmed with a home blood-glucose meter.

An rt-CGM can be used in conjunction with an insulin pump by establishing communication between the two devices. One of the primary purposes is to suspend insulin pumping when low glucose is detected. This is especially useful while sleeping but also in other situations like driving or other activities where hypoglycemia could be dangerous.

The next iteration in this technology is to program the insulin pump to adjust the insulin infusion based on rt-CGM results. This is called an artificial pancreas. On September 28, 2016, the FDA approved the first hybrid closed loop system, the Medtronic's MiniMed 670G System, intended to automatically monitor blood sugar and adjust basal insulin doses in people with type 1 diabetes.

Do these newer technologies improve glycemic control or prevent hypoglycemia? A meta-analysis done by a team from Johns Hopkins University and published in the *Annals of Internal Medicine* in 2012 examines this question.[55] The authors concluded:

> *For glycemic control, rt-CGM is superior to SMBG [self-monitored blood glucose] and sensor-augmented insulin pumps are superior to MDI [multiple dose injection] and SMBG without increasing the risk for hypoglycemia.*

Glycemic control as measured by HbA1c was better with rt-CGM, compared with SMBG, in children with T1DM, according to a meta-analysis titled "Systematic review and meta-analysis of the effectiveness of continuous glucose monitoring (CGM) on glucose control in diabetes."[56] The results of a 2011 randomized controlled trial by Battelino et al. on the effect of CGM monitoring on hypoglycemia, showed that in both children and adults with T1DM, the time per day spent in hypoglycemia was significantly shorter in the continuous-monitoring group (rt-CGM) than it was in the control group, and there was a concomitant decrease in HbA1c.[57]

Measuring, Tracking, and Establishing Glucose Profiles

Self-monitored blood-glucose measurements should be recorded and reviewed in a log before every dose of medication or insulin, and the log should be taken with you on visits to your doctor. This can be a simple row and column table on paper, or you can download a free blood-glucose and ketone-tracker sheet from the About This Site/ Resources section on ketogenic-diet-resource.com. The log should be used as an interactive tool to help determine any corrections needed to medications, insulin, or diet. This will help you improve blood-glucose control over the longer term.

Over the years, Dr. Runyan has seen patients report high blood-sugar results but fail to take any corrective actions, despite having been instructed how to do so. Worse yet, others fail to regularly measure their blood sugars. Typically, these are the patients who will have diabetic complications down the road. Knowing the misery that awaits them in the future, Dr. Runyan has been both frustrated and saddened. It's difficult to understand why some patients are unwilling to participate in their own care. Measuring blood-sugar levels solely for the purpose of documenting them is not very helpful. Instead, results of blood-sugar measurements should be used to make adjustments to treatment (diet, exercise, or medications) as you aim for your target blood-sugar level.

Measuring blood glucose is not difficult, and instructions are included with each glucose meter. Here are some general guidelines for testing your own blood-glucose levels. Make sure the skin is clean and free of food, glucose, and dirt. We suggest three locations on the fingers to prick with the lancet for better results. Use either the top of the fingers between the nail and first joint or between the first and middle joint. Avoid pricking over any joint.

The other location is on either side of the pad of each finger. Either side of the pad of each finger will yield blood readily, and there will be less discomfort compared with using the pad itself as is often incorrectly taught. Sometimes the thumb has thicker skin and should be avoided if it does not yield satisfactory results. Use locations and a lancet penetration depth that yields enough blood for your meter but is not painful.

Also, be aware that each finger has many potential areas to prick for blood-glucose or ketone measurements. Some glucose meters have a special lancet device for pricking the forearm, however, readings from this location will be less accurate and are therefore not recommended. Using the recommended locations with the correct depth of lancet insertion will provide accurate results with minimal discomfort. lancet insertion depths are adjustable on a five-level depth scale on most lancet devices.

Times and Reasons to Measure Blood Sugar

Note that most of these reasons are appropriate for those who take insulin or diabetic medications. If a ketogenic diet is followed closely and only insulin-sensitizing medications are used, the great majority of the those with T2DM will not require insulin therapy. Insulin therapy in T2DM is indicated for those who have had T2DM for many years, have low blood insulin levels, and do not have adequate blood sugar control. Giving insulin to those with T2DM with pre-existing hyperinsulinemia will increase the risk of the many previously mentioned diseases associated with T2DM including cardiovascular disease, heart attack, stroke, cancer, and Alzheimer's disease.

> Anytime you don't feel right and need to determine if that symptom is due to hypoglycemia.

> Upon rising, a fasting measurement is used to determine the correct evening or bedtime long-acting insulin (for T1DM or insulin-requiring T2DM) or whether the oral diabetes medications, if any, are at the correct dose. It can also detect the dawn phenomenon: an elevation in blood sugar due to the normal early morning rise in growth hormone and cortisol secretion in the setting of inadequate beta-cell insulin secretion.

> Before each meal, as this is used to determine the correct rapid acting or regular mealtime insulin dose (for T1DM or insulin-requiring T2DM) or whether any oral diabetes medications are at the correct dose, or to determine appropriate adjustments to your ketogenic diet. The insulin dose before meals is the sum of the insulin needed for the meal itself, plus or minus a corrective

insulin dose, if any. This will be reviewed in more detail in chapter 10. For those not taking any medications, elevated blood sugar can be addressed with reduced carbohydrate and/or protein specifically or with less food in general, or with exercise.

> For those not using insulin, check your two-hour postprandial blood glucose on some occasions. This will give you information about the balance between your medication and diet, or how your diet alone affects your blood sugar. This value should be close to your target blood-glucose level.

> After rapid-acting or regular insulin duration of action has ended, as this can vary from one individual to another and from one injection site to another. The duration of action of insulin can be determined by measuring blood glucose every thirty minutes after mealtime insulin injection. This will also be reviewed in more detail in chapter 10.

> Before going to bed, in case you need to correct with rapid-acting insulin or with adjustments in diet the following day or with glucose tablet(s) if blood sugar is low.

> Before and periodically while driving a car or operating heavy machinery or when engaged in any activity where you or others could be injured in the event of your having hypoglycemia. Note: this primarily applies to those taking insulin or sulfonylurea or glinide oral diabetes medications.

> Before and during long-term endurance exercise and after exercise as this will help determine how different types, intensities and durations of exercise affect your blood sugar and help determine your need for changes in diet, insulin and medications. Remember, physical activities such as cutting grass, cleaning house, and gardening, count as exercise as far as your blood sugar is concerned.

> During the night, if hypoglycemia at night is a problem for you. A real-time continuous glucose monitor is also helpful in alerting you to nighttime hypoglycemia.

➤ After a correction dose of rapid-acting insulin at the time you have determined to be the duration of action.

It's advisable to conduct a full blood-glucose profile as outlined in in the steps above for the entire day for several days in a row before your doctor visits. Blood-sugar control can change for many reasons, so it's a good idea to conduct a full blood-glucose profile periodically as well. That's the nature of having diabetes. If you're not regularly checking your blood-glucose profile, then you may have either unforeseen elevated HbA1c or an increased number or severity of hypoglycemic episodes. For those on multiple insulin injections or insulin pump therapy, the glucose profile should be a daily routine.

Please don't panic and throw up your hands in the air thinking that you have to check your blood sugars ten times each day. The number of daily blood-sugar measurements necessary to obtain and maintain optimal blood-glucose control will vary from one person to the next. In general, those taking insulin or other medications that have the potential to cause hypoglycemia (sulfonylurea or glinide oral diabetes medications) will need more frequent blood-glucose measurements. That said, once you're used to measuring blood glucose frequently, and you realize how much better your blood-glucose values are because of it, we suspect you won't mind. On days when you are not measuring your blood-glucose profile, the number of blood-sugar measurements will be fewer.

Finally, even if your blood-glucose meter has electronic memory and can send your readings to your and/or your doctor's computer, it is important to keep a written log of your blood glucose, ketone, and HbA1c readings, and take notes that may help you make future adjustments in diet, exercise and other corrective measures. Your notes should include the amount and type of exercise, any symptoms of hypoglycemia, the number of glucose tablets taken to correct it, and stressful or unusual situations that might affect your blood sugars, like exercise, illness, travel, or a new job.

You can download and print the data sheet offered at the bottom of the About This Site/Resources page of ketogenic-diet-resource.com, use a spreadsheet program, or make your own log. The Wisconsin Diabetes Prevention website offers a useful log book you can download and print,[58] or you can search for "blood-sugar log" in Google or Bing and choose the one you like.

Blood-Glucose Targets

"Target" blood glucose is the desired average blood glucose for a particular individual. Factors to consider when determining a target include motivation, age, diabetic complications, and financial and social support.

When we talk about target blood glucose, we must include both short-term and long-term goals. The short-term blood-glucose target is largely determined by the individual's current level of glycemic control. For example, if a person with poorly controlled diabetes (HbA1c of 10%, roughly equivalent to an average blood glucose of 240 mg/dL (13.3 mmol/L)) were to start a strict ketogenic diet with 30 grams of carbohydrate per day, there is a chance that this person could develop symptoms of hypoglycemia at levels of blood glucose that measure in the normal range.

The ketogenic diet can result in a rapid reduction in blood glucose during the first few days, even before keto-adaptation occurs, especially if diabetes medications are not reduced during the process. This person may develop the symptoms of hypoglycemia once blood glucose falls to, say, 100–120 mg/dL (5.6–6.7 mmol/L), which is above normal. The poorer the glycemic control (or the higher the initial HbA1c), the more likely that symptoms of hypoglycemia will be experienced. The exact reasons for this long-recognized phenomenon are not well characterized. As glycemic control improves over time, symptoms of hypoglycemia will occur at lower levels of blood glucose.

In order to minimize the likelihood of hypoglycemia in people with higher blood sugars, daily dietary-carbohydrate intake can be gradually dropped over time while insulin and/or oral diabetes medications are reduced. This should be discussed with your doctor, who can help you determine which medications should be reduced first, the rate at which to reduce them, and which can be discontinued.

The short-term blood glucose target would also be gradually lowered over time. The short-term goal is used to help determine insulin and medication dose adjustments with the help of your physician. For the motivated person with fairly well controlled diabetes (HbA1c of 6%, roughly equivalent to an average blood glucose of 126 mg/dL (7.0 mmol/L)), starting a strict ketogenic diet with 30 grams of carbohydrate with a near normal blood-glucose target would be a reasonable starting point.

The time needed to reach the long-term blood-glucose target will vary from person to person. It may take several months or longer to reach that goal by adjusting insulin doses and medications while avoiding hypoglycemia. It is more important to eventually reach your target blood glucose than to get frustrated because it hasn't been reached in some arbitrary time frame.

The ketogenic diet has the potential to rapidly reduce the need for insulin and medications in those with T2DM who have normal insulin-secreting capacity. It makes much more sense to work with your physician to decrease medications and insulin in response to a reduction in dietary carbohydrates rather than continue to consume carbohydrates to accommodate the medications and insulin.

If the initial blood-glucose target is not obtainable due to hypoglycemia, inability to follow the ketogenic diet, or inability to monitor blood glucose frequently enough, or for any other reason, then you should aim for a somewhat higher blood-glucose target—but still aim for as low of a target as you can manage safely without having hypoglycemia.

Neither the ketogenic diet nor glycemic control of diabetes is an all-or-nothing proposition. The goal is to achieve the lowest average blood glucose that you can while avoiding hypoglycemia. For example, if you can follow a 75 gram/day carbohydrate non-ketogenic diet and achieve an average blood glucose of 100 mg/dL without hypoglycemia, and that's better than your previous markers, then your health will be much improved. Your specific blood-glucose and HbA1c targets should be discussed with your doctor as you review your blood-glucose profile and current HbA1c results.

Blood-Sugar Reference Tables

The tables for fasting and postprandial blood-sugar ranges below are meant to provide a frame of reference for target blood-glucose and HbA1c discussions with your physician.

Fasting Blood Sugar Recommendations

Fasting blood sugar is a measurement of your blood sugar after not eating for eight to twelve hours. This test is normally included with a comprehensive metabolic profile (CMP) test. Fasting blood sugars are evaluated as follows by the American Diabetes Association[59] and the American College of Clinical Endocrinologists.[60]

Fasting Blood Glucose: Diagnostic Criteria		
	ADA	AACE
Normal blood sugar: range:	<100 mg/dL	<100 mg/dL
Prediabetic range:	101–126 mg/dL	101–126 mg /dL
Diabetic range:	≥126 mg/dL (7.0 mmol/L)	≥126 mg/dL (7.0 mmol/L)

Postprandial Blood Sugar Recommendations

Postprandial blood sugar is a measurement of your blood sugar one to two hours after a meal. Postprandial blood sugars are evaluated as follows by the American Diabetes Association and the American College of Clinical Endocrinologists.

Postprandial Diagnostic Chart and Treatment Goals			
	For healthy persons	Goals for persons with diabetes	
		ADA	AACE
Blood sugars before meals:	<100 mg/dL	70–130 mg/dL	<110 mg/dL
Blood sugars two hours after meal:	<120 mg/dL	<180 mg/dL	<140 mg/dL

A study titled "Variation of interstitial glucose measurements assessed by continuous glucose monitors in healthy, non-diabetic individuals" by Beck, et al., followed 74 healthy children, adolescents, and adults and found the average interstitial (similar to blood glucose) glucose over 24 hours was 98 mg/dl (5.4 mM). The diet of these individuals was not controlled or measured and it's likely they were not on a low carbohydrate diet. Average blood glucose would probably be lower on a low carbohydrate diet, but to date, there is no similar study data to confirm this. However, these individuals at the time of the study did not have metabolic syndrome, so the average glucose of 98 mg/dl is likely a healthy reading and would be a reasonable target that those with diabetes can aim.

Hypoglycemia: Symptoms and Treatment

Hypoglycemia is usually accompanied by one or more of the signs or symptoms shown below. If a type 1 or type 2 diabetic using sulfonylurea or glinide medications or insulin therapy develop hypoglycemia, the normal counter-regulatory response of the pancreatic alpha cells to secrete glucagon is impaired. This results in loss of the normal signal to the liver to create glucose via glycogenolysis or gluconeogenesis when it is needed to raise blood glucose.

Hypoglycemia causes a cascade of signaling that stimulates the release of adrenalin (epinephrine and norepinephrine) and acetylcholine. These neurotransmitters and hormones are responsible for many of the signs and symptoms of hypoglycemia. These symptoms serve as warning signs to seek out food/glucose to correct the problem.

Common Symptoms of Hypoglycemia

Symptoms of hypoglycemia should be treated immediately with glucose in the form of tablets or liquid, regardless of the availability of a glucose meter or blood-glucose reading or which diet the patient is following.

- Confusion
- Nervousness
- Irritability
- Stubbornness
- Anxiety or panic
- Nasty behavior
- Blurred vision
- Double vision
- Unable to read or comprehend text
- Seeing spots or lights
- Visual hallucinations
- Increased hunger
- Nausea
- Restlessness
- Tiredness
- Weakness
- Rapid heartbeat
- Pounding heartbeat
- Ringing or buzzing in ears
- Sweating, feeling hot
- Sweating, feeling cold
- Headache
- Nightmares
- Appearing pale
- Dilated pupils

- Involuntary eye movement
- Slurred speech
- Convulsions/seizures
- Fainting
- Dizziness
- Lightheadedness
- Dizziness on standing
- Uncontrolled limb movements
- Clumsiness
- Difficulty walking
- Drops objects
- Inappropriate laughter
- Numbness anywhere on the body
- Tremors of hands
- Insomnia
- Awakening from sleep
- Shouting while awake or asleep
- Coma

In a person with insulin-requiring T2DM who has had numerous hypoglycemic episodes in the recent past, symptoms of hypoglycemia are diminished due to a reduced sympathetic nervous system response to epinephrine/norepinephrine. This is called *hypoglycemia unawareness* but, more accurately, is an impaired awareness of hypoglycemia with reduced symptoms.[61] This is a problem for persons with diabetes because it leads to a vicious cycle of recurrent hypoglycemia and increases the risk of severe hypoglycemia six to twenty-five fold. Severe hypoglycemia increases the risk of death from hypoglycemia, an event which occurs in up to 10% of persons with diabetes. Thus, avoiding hypoglycemia is very important, particularly if the symptoms are fewer than previously experienced.

When patients are hypoglycemic, it is common for them to go into a "panic mode." This often results in excessive consumption of sweets with subsequent hyperglycemia, and is one of the reasons why hypoglycemia is a factor in failure to achieve successful blood-sugar control.[62] To avoid sugar overdosing and hyperglycemia, it is preferable to use pure glucose tablets or gel (sold in grocery stores, pharmacies and online) because these products will resolve the hypoglycemia very quickly. Table sugar will work in a pinch, but it's not the best option since it contains sucrose composed of fructose and glucose bound together. The better solution is to keep a supply of glucose tablets or liquid close at hand. If you find yourself without them, anything sweetened with sugar will also work (e.g. non-diet cola, fruit juice, or candies like Smarties® or SweeTARTS®).

If you suspect you may be hypoglycemic but are not sure, measure blood glucose and treat accordingly to bring it up to your target using the appropriate number of glucose tablets; keep in mind that each tablet contains four grams of glucose. It is also appropriate to take glucose tablets or sugar for suspected hypoglycemia if your glucose meter is not immediately available.

Since a normal bloodstream only contains about five grams of glucose, you can see that hypoglycemia can be corrected with one or two tablets. It will take ten to fifteen minutes for the symptoms of hypoglycemia to resolve after consuming the glucose. If symptoms have not resolved in ten to fifteen minutes, check your blood sugar to determine if your symptoms are due to hypoglycemia or, if your meter is not available, take additional glucose or sweets. If symptoms persist, seek medical attention. Using glucose tablets does not take into account further absorption of injected insulin or the effects of oral diabetes medications, so a small snack containing protein will help prevent another drop in your blood glucose during subsequent hours.

Reactive Hypoglycemia

A study titled "Acute effects on insulin sensitivity and diurnal metabolic profiles of a high-sucrose compared with a high-starch diet" showed that

consuming a diet with 50% carbohydrates as sugar resulted in abnor-
mally low blood-glucose values two to three hours after each meal.[63]
This is called reactive hypoglycemia, and it is caused by an exaggerated
release of insulin in response to a large spike in blood-sugar levels as
a result of a meal high in refined carbohydrates. Common symptoms
include irritability, hunger, weakness, shakiness, sleepiness, sweating,
lightheadedness, anxiety and confusion occurring within two to four
hours of the last meal. Reactive hypoglycemia is more common in
people who are insulin resistant. Although many people experience
it, they may not be aware of the cause.

Most individuals who depend on carbohydrates for fuel learn to eat
or drink something high in carbohydrate to relieve their symptoms. In
fact, people with reactive hypoglycemia are often advised to snack on
something with carbohydrate every few hours in order to "keep the
blood sugar up." This does temporarily prevent the unpleasant symptoms
of hypoglycemia, but it does nothing to correct the underlying cause
of the low blood sugar in the first place. In fact, all this strategy does is
perpetuate a disastrous blood-sugar roller coaster. And, over time, the
usual food choices of juice, soda, glucose tablets or other quick-acting
carbohydrates can lead to weight gain due to elevated insulin levels
and extra carbohydrate consumption needed to relieve symptoms.

Many of the unpleasant symptoms of reactive hypoglycemia are the
result of perceived glucose deprivation by the brain. Because the brain
has very low glucose reserves, it needs a constant supply of glucose from
the bloodstream. In the carbohydrate-adapted individual, that blood
glucose has to be replenished from food sources every few hours. When
a person follows a ketogenic diet, fuel flow is not a problem. Insulin
levels are low and insulin sensitivity is normal or improving, which
allows the use of fatty acids and ketones as the primary fuels. Since
there is a large supply of these nutrients available in adipose (body fat)
tissue stores, reactive hypoglycemia does not typically happen when
one is on a ketogenic diet.

Hyperglycemia and Glycation Damage

Hyperglycemia is a condition in which excessive amounts of glucose build up in blood plasma due to either a lack of insulin or a lack of response to insulin from body tissues. A diabetic with uncontrolled blood sugars may have two to ten times the normal amount of glucose in his or her bloodstream. Excursions of blood sugar that exceed normal levels are the main cause of diabetic complications.[64]

The damage of hyperglycemia is a function of uncontrolled amounts of blood sugar being processed through cellular energy pathways. The influx of large amounts of glucose into cells increases production of reactive oxygen species (ROS), volatile compounds that can kill cells via chemical damage to cellular structures.

Elevations of ROS or "free radicals" are associated with the progression of glycation damage. Glycation is a process in which excess blood glucose bonds or "sticks" to various protein molecules in body tissues. The bonding of sugar molecules causes an impairment of the glycated tissue and, eventually, causes extensive damage and loss of function through the formation of advanced glycation end products (AGEs). To get a good idea of how glycation works, imagine what would happen if you were to rub maple syrup on your hands and then try to fold clothes or type on a keyboard.

Measures of Glycation Damage

Measures of glycation damage are used as an estimate of hyperglycemia over time. The longer blood sugar is elevated, the more likely glycation damage will occur. A test called hemoglobin A1c (or simply HbA1c) measures the level of hemoglobin (a protein found in red blood cells) that becomes glycated when exposed to blood glucose. The longer and higher blood glucose remains above normal, the larger the percentage of hemoglobin molecules that become glycated. Measuring the amount of glycated hemoglobin gives an average of blood-sugar levels over the past two to three months.

The composition of one's diet is closely tied to average blood-glucose values and, therefore, HbA1c results. A study done at the Human Nutrition Research Centre at the University of Newcastle upon Tyne in the United Kingdom demonstrates the effect of starch and sugar in the diet on blood glucose in eight healthy volunteers who received a standard diet providing 55% of energy as carbohydrate, 35% as fat and 10% as protein.

After a starch-rich meal, blood glucose peaks one hour after the meal but does not return to the pre-meal value until the following morning. After a sugar-rich meal, blood glucose peaks one hour after each meal and then drops below baseline two to three hours after each meal. This is an example of reactive hypoglycemia.

The important point here is that the study shows that glucose levels are elevated after meals and overnight. Hence, glycation damage is more likely to occur. And even though these glucose elevations after meals are temporary, they cause an elevation in average blood sugars over time. In addition, hemoglobin is not the only protein that becomes glycated during these episodes of elevated blood sugar. Numerous other proteins can be damaged by glycation. A review paper by Goldin et al. describes the consequences of glycation that occur in patients with diabetes.[65] Glycation is involved in the complications of diabetes, such as diabetic nephropathy (kidney disease and kidney failure),[66] neuropathy (nerve damage, numbness of skin, loss of body perception, Charcot foot, and muscle weakness)[67] and retinopathy (retinal hemorrhage, vitreous hemorrhage, neovascularization, and blindness).[68]

And glycation damage is not limited to those with diabetes. It occurs any time blood glucose and HbA1c are persistently higher than normal, especially when inflammation is also present.

Hemoglobin A1c Test Accuracy

Physicians order glycated hemoglobin A1c tests every three to six months to monitor patient blood-glucose control with the idea that it's a rough measure of the average blood glucose over the previous two to three months. Having a substitute for average blood glucose helps physicians monitor current blood-glucose control in patients who will not check their blood glucose on a regular basis.

Although studies have suggested that there is a correlation between HbA1c and average blood glucose, and that HbA1c results can serve as a substitute for average blood glucose, self-monitored blood-glucose readings are more accurate. HbA1c test results can vary greatly from one person to another, even if people have the same average blood glucose. For example, in a 1993 paper titled "The effect of intensive treatment of diabetes on the development and progression of long-term complications in insulin-dependent diabetes mellitus," diabetics with mean plasma glucose of 214 mg/dL (11.9 mmol/L) had HbA1c results ranging from 6.2% to 12.4%, while diabetics with mean plasma glucose of 115 mg/dL (6.4 mmol/L) had HbA1c results ranging from 5.4% to 8.6%.[69]

Changes in HbA1c results over time is a useful measure of changing blood-sugar control because average blood glucose is highly correlated with individual HbA1c results. Hence, HbA1c can be of value in monitoring your progress after making a change in diet (say, changing to the ketogenic diet) or after making a change in insulin (type or dose) or other diabetes medications. You can check your HbA1c more frequently (every three to four weeks initially) by having your own HbA1c meter. The A1c Now+ meter by Chek Diagnostics is one such meter. Keep in mind that readings from any meter will have the same value and limitations as laboratory HbA1c tests. The best way to monitor blood-glucose control is to measure your own glucose profile using your home glucose meter.

Fructosamine

Fructosamine is a glycated molecule formed from the bonding of fructose to protein-carrier molecules in the blood (mostly albumin). Similar to HbA1c tests, a fructosamine test is designed to measure average blood glucose, but since albumin decays after fourteen to twenty-one days, the fructosamine test reflects average blood-sugar concentrations over the previous two to three weeks, instead of months as indicated by an HbA1c.

The fructosamine test has been available through laboratories since the early 1980s. It's useful for monitoring a dietary or medication adjustment to correct blood glucose quickly, especially during pregnancy. It's also useful in patients with genetic defects that result in an abnormal structure within red blood cell hemoglobin molecules where the hemoglobin A1c test results might be misleading.

The interpretation of fructosamine depends upon the individual's age and sex. The table below gives the diagnostic ranges. Because of the significant overlap in these ranges, the relative change in fructosamine over time is more valuable than the absolute number.

Population	Fructosamine range
Non-diabetic individuals	175 to 280 mmol/L
Diabetics with controlled blood sugars	210 to 421 mmol/L
Diabetics with uncontrolled blood sugars	268 to 870 mmol/L

In patients with shortened red blood cell lifespans, fructosamine is thought to be more reliable than the HbA1c test.[70] These conditions include kidney disease, liver disease, hemolytic anemia, HIV, iron-deficiency anemia, and aplastic anemia.

Troubleshooting Elevated Blood Glucose

Lowering blood sugar and increasing ketone levels can be difficult, even when following a strict ketogenic diet. Here are some points to consider if you are having trouble getting your baseline blood-sugar levels to drop.

➤ *Physical stress*: Diabetes is a metabolic source of stress. Just trying to control your blood sugar becomes a source of worry and stress-generated aberrations.

➤ *Mental stress*: Excess emotional stress can increase levels of cortisol, a hormone that can increase blood sugar. Find ways to decrease emotional and mental stress. Try yoga, prayer, meditation, or art projects or doing something that you love that absorbs your attention and takes your mind off your health.

> *Medications*: Some medications such as barbiturates, diuretics, catecholamines, and antipsychotics can increase blood sugar. Talk to your primary care physician about alternatives if this becomes an issue. A list of 390 drugs that can affect your blood sugar is available at www.diabetesincontrol.com.[71]

> *Protein consumption*: It is very easy to "overeat" protein if food intake is not tracked via a food scale and log. At each meal, most people only need a serving of meat about the size of a deck of playing cards. To test, try lowering daily protein intake by ten grams. In other words, eat about 1.25 ounces less protein each day.

> *Hidden carbs*: Read labels and count every carbohydrate in food, drinks, and supplements. Sugar alcohols and hidden fillers can cause blood-sugar spikes and interfere with ketosis for some people.

> *Low thyroid function*: Check with your doctor on your thyroid status.

> *Carbohydrate intake on food labels*: Food labels do not provide accurate measures of carbohydrate. Food manufacturers can list zero carbohydrates for up to 0.5 grams of carbohydrate per serving.

> *Vitamins, fish oil, herbal supplements*: These can have hidden carbs. In addition, taking large amounts of fish oil can drive up blood sugar. You may have to eliminate your supplements for several days while monitoring your blood sugar. Then reintroduce the supplements one at a time to determine which might be the source of trouble.

> *Caffeine intake*: Drinking caffeinated coffee or sugar-free cocoa or eating dark chocolate and other foods containing caffeine can drive up blood sugar.

> *Caloric intake*: Use a Base Metabolic Rate (BMR) calorie calculator to find the recommended caloric intake for your goal weight and adjust your caloric intake to match.[72]

> *Exercise*: In persons with T2DM not taking insulin, sulfonylureas, or glinide medications, moderate exercise has little immediate effect on blood sugar. In contrast, vigorous exercise can raise blood sugar during and immediately after exercise. This is a normal stress response designed to supply glucose and fatty acids to exercising muscles. Over time, both moderate and vigorous exercise reduce blood sugar and insulin levels. Normally, insulin would be secreted by the pancreas to correct blood sugar after exercise, but in those with diabetes this response may be delayed.

> *Micronutrients*: Deficiencies of micronutrients such as magnesium and chromium can be detrimental to blood-sugar control. Taking at least a basic multi-vitamin/multi-mineral each day is recommended. Vitamin D levels should also be checked and optimized. See supplement recommendations in appendix A.

> *Colds, flu, and other illnesses*: Fighting off viral or bacterial infections, like colds or the flu, will result in elevated blood sugars. In addition, most cold medications are laced with some type of sugar. It's a good idea to search out cold and flu medications that are carbohydrate free and stock up. Ask your pharmacist to assist you.

> *Menstrual cycles*: Women should be aware that the onset of menstruation also elevates blood sugar for a few days.

> *Insulin resistance*: As we age, most of us eating a standard high-carbohydrate diet develop some sort of insulin resistance resulting in high insulin levels and eventually chronically high glucose. It takes time for this condition to reverse itself once a ketogenic diet is started. Months or years is not an uncommon time frame, especially when excess body fat persists.

> *Age in general*: Younger people will generally respond better to dietary changes with faster drops in blood sugar and higher ketone levels, often within days of starting the diet. Older people will find this process takes longer.

> *Consistency of meal macronutrients:* It is important to keep the macronutrient (protein, fat, and carbs) amounts and ratios consistent at each meal from day to day. This makes predicting insulin dose needs and blood glucose response much more consistent from day to day.

Monitoring Ketone Levels

When following a ketogenic diet, monitoring urine, blood, or breath ketones can provide useful information about whether you are in a state of nutritional ketosis. Why is this important? Monitoring ketones can provide some assurance that you are following the ketogenic diet correctly and that a state of nutritional ketosis has been achieved.

Measuring urine ketones is the least expensive way to monitor nutritional ketosis. Bayer Ketostix is one such product. Ketone strips detect acetoacetate in urine and range from trace (<5 mg/dL) to large (160 mg/dL). When beginning the ketogenic diet, it may take several days for urine ketones to rise above trace amounts. Moderate to large urine ketones (40–160 mg/dL) are consistent with nutritional ketosis. It is important to keep in mind that the absence of darker pink or purple on your urine test strips does not necessarily mean your body isn't generating ketones. Many factors can affect the concentration of acetoacetate in the urine throughout the day. After months on a ketogenic diet, many individuals can be in nutritional ketosis yet have only trace urine ketones due to improved renal reabsorption of ketones.[73] While in a state of nutritional ketosis, urine ketones could be temporarily at a trace level if your water intake is higher than average. Alternatively, urine-ketone levels could be higher (160 mg/dL) because of low fluid intake or fluid loss from sweating, vomiting, or diarrhea. Dehydration acts to concentrate urine, which increases urine-ketone concentration. Persistently negative urine ketones can also reflect an absence of nutritional ketosis due to excessive intakes of carbohydrate or protein or both.

Ketones measured in urine were noted to be reflective of changes in serum, and this led to the adoption of urine-ketone measurement as a standard method for determining the degree of ketosis induced by a ketogenic diet. But blood ketones are still a valuable tool. For example, if you have had positive urine ketones in the past, and if, without a change in your ketogenic diet, your urine ketones become persistently negative, measuring blood ketones can help determine the cause. When you have negative urine ketones but your blood ketones are in excess of 0.5 mM, the kidneys may have improved their ability to retain ketones—to the point that measuring urine ketones will no longer be a useful test for you. However, if you have negative urine ketones and your blood ketones are less than 0.5 mM, this means that the ketones actually are low, indicating that you are not in nutritional ketosis. Your diet has changed enough to stop ketosis, and you should reassess your carbohydrate and protein intake.

A blood-ketone meter, like Abbott Laboratories' Precision Xtra, measures the concentration of a ketone called beta-hydroxybutyrate (BHOB) in millimoles per liter (mmole/liter or mM). Nutritional ketosis is defined as having levels of blood BHOB in the range of 0.5–3 mM per the recommendation of Jeff Volek, RD, PhD, and Stephen Phinney, MD, PhD. Note that blood-ketone levels vary during the course of the day, with higher readings in the afternoon.[74]

Whether it is better to have a blood BHOB concentration closer to 3 mM than to 0.5 mM when treating diabetes is not clear at this point. Based on studies of fasting humans,[75] the brain oxidation of ketones increases linearly as the blood-ketone levels increase to 4 mM. Brain oxidation of ketones levels off as blood-ketone levels increase above 4 mM total ketone-body concentration. A total ketone-body concentration of 4 mM corresponds to a BHOB concentration of 3 mM. Thus, it is theoretically possible that the brain could be protected from hypoglycemia, at least partially, by having blood BHOB concentrations closer to 3 mM than to 0.5 mM. This needs to be studied in persons with T2DM on a ketogenic diet. The primary determinate of blood BHOB concentration is the degree of carbohydrate restriction: fewer dietary carbohydrates translates to more ketones. The secondary determinate is dietary-protein intake: less protein intake translates to more ketones. Although there is no dietary requirement for carbohydrates, you do need protein in a range of 1.0–1.5 grams/kg BW/day. Also, remember that there are foods that are beneficial and nutrient dense that contain small amounts of carbohydrate and should be included in a ketogenic diet. A ketogenic diet for diabetes should be low in carbohydrates but not necessarily absent of carbohydrates.

The Ketonix meter measures acetone in the breath. Acetone is a spontaneous by-product of acetoacetate, one of the ketones produced by the liver during nutritional ketosis. Ketonix was developed by an engineer in Sweden, Michel Lundell, who wanted an easier method to monitor his own nutritional ketosis for treatment of epilepsy. It is a one-time expense, but it can be used hundreds of times, making it quite cost effective. Ketonix is also easy and convenient to use since you simply exhale into the device, and no blood or urine is needed. It has not been independently tested against blood or urine measurements, so each individual needs to make his or her own correlation between the percentage (0–100%) readout and the personal therapeutic goals. By way of disclosure, a Ketonix device was gifted to Dr. Runyan by Michel Lundell. Dr. Runyan has posted his results using this device on his blog.[76]

In the next chapter, we will examine diabetic medications and supplements. We include information on how they work and why they are prescribed, including whether they are compatible with a ketogenic diet.

9

Medications and Supplements

Individuals taking any of the medications discussed in this chapter should check with their doctors or qualified health providers who are knowledgeable about ketogenic diets before beginning the diet. Dosages may need to be adjusted, and there may be contraindications or interactions with other prescribed drugs, so it's very important to involve your prescribing physician before you start. A paper by Triplett discusses the drug interactions possible with medications commonly used to treat diabetes and is a recommended source of information.[77]

In addition, various nutritional supplements can either interfere with or intensify the effect of hypoglycemic drugs. In particular, caution should be exercised when combining diabetes medications with nutritional supplements that also lower blood sugar. The list below includes the nutritional supplements most likely to be problematic. Taking these supplements with hypoglycemic drugs can increase the risk of low blood sugar, especially when multiple supplements are taken.

- Alpha Lipoic Acid
- Bilberry
- Berberine
- Chromium
- Cinnamon
- Garlic
- Gingko Biloba
- Ginseng
- Green Tea Catechins

- Melatonin
- Resveratrol
- St. John's Wort
- Vanadium

Another supplement interaction to be aware of is that of fish oil. For some people with prediabetes and diabetes, taking large amounts of fish oil can increase blood sugar[78] and be detrimental to glycemic control.[79]

Hypoglycemic Drugs on the Ketogenic Diet

Let's now review oral and subcutaneously injected medications used for glycemic control in T2DM. When a properly formulated ketogenic diet, weight loss, and regular exercise are not enough to lower blood sugars to your target, then one or more oral or subcutaneously injected medications, including insulin, can be added. Remember that for those with T2DM, insulin should be the last pharmaceutical agent employed in the treatment of hyperglycemia. Ideally, it should be reserved for those with an inability to secrete normal amounts of insulin.

If insulin was administered to the vast majority of those with T2DM who are insulin resistant and make normal or above normal amounts of insulin, the negative health conditions associated with T2DM (cardiovascular disease, heart attack, stroke, high blood pressure, metabolic syndrome, abnormal blood lipids, obesity, cancer, and numerous other conditions) would be more likely to occur even if blood sugar levels are improved with insulin administration.

Every drug used to treat a medical condition has potential adverse effects. These effects range from minor symptoms to major life-threatening and fatal reactions. Therefore, using all available information, a judgment must be made concerning the risk-to-benefit ratio. Doctors prescribing medication try to minimize this ratio. Largely, this is an assessment of whether the benefits of a medication outweigh its potential risks. You can appreciate how difficult it is to predict this for a specific individual.

Websites such as rxlist.com, drugs.com, and many others provide patients and physicians with access to a great deal of information on medication benefits, risks, and side effects. We will be discussing benefits and risks for most of the classes of hypoglycemic medications in the following sections. Although there is extensive information available about these medications, but we certainly cannot cover it all, so we will focus on the more important points. Our goal in this section is to give you a "pros and cons" overview of the available hypoglycemic medications so that you can make an informed choice if your physician suggests that you begin taking any of them. We will start with metformin, which is usually the first medication prescribed after a diagnosis of type 2 diabetes.

Metformin

Metformin is generally recognized as first-line drug treatment for T2DM due to its favorable mechanism of action, effectiveness and low side-effect profile. It was first introduced to the United Kingdom in 1958, Canada in 1972, and the United States in 1995, and it is now believed to be the most widely prescribed antidiabetic drug in the world. It is used for the following insulin resistant states:

- Type 2 diabetes mellitus
- Prediabetes
- Obesity with insulin resistance
- Metabolic syndrome
- Polycystic ovarian syndrome (PCOS)

Although a switch to a ketogenic diet may be all that is necessary to resolve insulin resistance, obesity/being overweight, or poor glycemic control, metformin may be appropriate during the transition or if there is difficulty being strict with the ketogenic diet. Metformin lowers blood glucose by decreasing liver-glucose production and improves insulin sensitivity by increasing cellular-glucose uptake and utilization. It has the following clinical advantages:

- Extensive experience with the medication
- No association with weight gain
- Does not cause hypoglycemia when administered alone
- Low cost

The disadvantages of adding Metformin to insulin include a possible increase in the likelihood of hypoglycemia, especially if the insulin dose is not appropriately reduced in response to switching to a ketogenic diet or adding metformin to an insulin regimen. In addition, a vitamin B12 deficiency can occur in 7% of those taking metformin as a long-term therapy, and there is a very small risk for lactic acidosis, especially if there is an underlying health factor such as heart failure or hypoxia.[80]

Metformin can also deplete vitamin B9 (folic acid). Gastrointestinal symptoms including nausea, diarrhea, and abdominal cramping. Starting at a low dose and increasing the dose slowly can minimize these GI side effects.

A recent observational study from the Swedish National Diabetes Register examined cardiovascular and all-cause mortality and the risk of lactic acidosis and infection in T2DM patients taking metformin compared with other oral hypoglycemic agents (OHA) or insulin. They concluded:

> Metformin showed lower risk than insulin for CVD and all-cause mortality and slightly lower risk for all-cause mortality compared with other OHA, in these 51,675 patients followed for 4 years. Patients with renal impairment showed no increased risk of CVD, all-cause mortality or acidosis/serious infection. In clinical practice, the benefits of metformin use clearly outbalance the risk of severe side effects.[81]

The glucose-lowering effectiveness of metformin is high in those who consume a diet high in carbohydrates. The expected HbA1c reduction is 1.0%–1.5%. Metformin is the lowest cost hypoglycemic medication. There is uniform agreement that the drug is the first-line hypoglycemic medication for T2DM. It's also compatible with a ketogenic diet. Overall, when a properly formulated ketogenic diet, weight loss, and regular exercise are not enough to lower blood sugars to your target, metformin is by far the safest and most effective medication currently available to treat pre-diabetes and T2DM.

Sulfonylureas

Sulfonylureas are the oldest class of oral hypoglycemic agents. The first-generation drugs include carbutamide, acetohexamide, chlorpropamide, tolbutamide, and tolazamide. The second generation of drugs in the class include glipizide, gliclazide, glibenclamide, glibornuride, gliquidone, glisoxepide, glyclopyramide, and glimepiride.

Sulfonylureas cause nonspecific glucose-independent stimulation of insulin release, meaning that insulin release is not related to current blood-glucose levels. Therefore, these drugs can result in excessive pancreatic insulin secretion, which can cause hypoglycemia, weight gain and an increase in the risk of developing cardiovascular disease and other previously mentioned negative health conditions associated with T2DM. These drugs can also deplete sodium and CoQ10, and, when combined with alcohol, first-generation sulfonylurea drugs (such as chlorpropramide) can cause facial flushing.

Obviously, there won't be many carbohydrates in a ketogenic meal to offset the unregulated insulin secretion from beta cells induced by sulfonylurea drugs. This can result in extended hypoglycemia, a potentially dangerous condition. Depending on the duration of action of the drug and the individual's level of kidney function, hypoglycemia can last for many hours. Hence, compatibility with a ketogenic diet is questionable. Use with caution, or avoid altogether, while following a ketogenic diet.

In the minority of those with T2DM, pancreatic insulin secretion is impaired due to long-standing insulin resistance and beta-cell exhaustion. Sulfonylureas stimulate insulin secretion that can exacerbate beta-cell dysfunction. A study by Takahashi et al. provides more details on this effect.[82] A recent retrospective cohort study by Pantalone et al.

concluded that "glipizide, glyburide and glimepiride are associated with an increased risk of overall mortality versus metformin."[83]

And in another 2014 study published in *Diabetes, Obesity and Metabolism* by Morgan et al., the authors concluded that "all-cause mortality was significantly increased in patients prescribed sulphonylurea compared with metformin monotherapy. Whilst residual confounding and confounding by indication may remain, this study indicates that first-line treatment with sulphonylurea monotherapy should be reconsidered."

Meglitinides (Glinides)

The three drugs in this class include repaglinide (Prandin), nateglinide (Starlix) and mitiglinide (Glufast in Japan). Their mechanism of action is the same as for sulfonylureas. Their duration of action is shorter and, thus, requires more frequent dosing. Side effects include weight gain and hypoglycemia.

While the potential for hypoglycemia is less compared with sulfonylureas, it is still a serious potential side effect that can be life-threatening. Presumably, hypoglycemia would be more marked on a ketogenic diet. The glucose-lowering effectiveness of meglitinides is modest. In those who consume carbohydrates, expected HbA1c reduction is 0.5%–1.0%. Cost of the drug is high when compared to metformin and sulfonylureas.

The glucose-independent stimulation of insulin release by meglitinides makes them more likely to cause a significant increase in the frequency and severity of hypoglycemic episodes, especially while following a ketogenic diet, so they should be used with great caution or avoided altogether.

Thiazolidinediones (TZDs)

The four drugs in this class include pioglitazone, rivoglitazone, rosiglitazone, and troglitazone. Thiazolidinediones are peroxisome proliferator-activated receptor (PPAR) gamma agonists with multiple actions that lead to improved insulin sensitivity. There are potential problems with medications in this class of oral hypoglycemic agents that must be weighed against potential benefits.

Rosiglitazone (Avandia) was put under selling restrictions in the United States and withdrawn from the market in Europe due to meta-analyses suggesting an increased risk of cardiovascular events. It was banned in the United Kingdom and India in 2010. In New Zealand, rosiglitazone was withdrawn from the market in April 2011. Upon re-evaluation of the 2013 study, Rosiglitazone evaluated for cardiovascular outcomes in oral agent combination therapy for type 2 diabetes (RECORD), the US Food and Drug Administration lifted restrictions.[84]

Sales of pioglitazone (Actos) were suspended in France and Germany after a study suggested it could raise the risk of bladder cancer.[85] Troglitazone (Rezulin) was withdrawn from the market due to an increased incidence of drug-induced hepatitis. Other side effects included weight gain, edema, congestive heart failure, bone fractures, increased LDL-C (rosiglitazone), and questionable increased risk of myocardial infarction shown in meta-analyses associated with rosiglitazone.[86]

The glucose-lowering potential is high for TZDs. In those who consume carbohydrates, the expected HbA1c reduction is 1.0%–1.5%. The cost of this drug is high when compared to metformin and sulfonylureas. The mechanism of action of thiazolidinediones is to improve insulin sensitivity. Thiazolidinediones do not independently cause hypoglycemia, making this class of hypoglycemic agents compatible with a ketogenic diet.

Glucagon-Like Peptide 1 (GLP-1) Agonists

These drugs enhance the action of glucagon-like peptide 1 (GLP-1), a beneficial intestinal hormone secreted in response to the presence of nutrients in the small intestine. GLP-1 stimulates insulin secretion while suppressing glucagon secretion. Such glucose-dependent action is particularly attractive because when plasma glucose is in the normal fasting range, GLP-1 no longer stimulates insulin that might lead to hypoglycemia. GLP-1 appears to restore glucose sensitivity of pancreatic beta cells. GLP-1 is also known to inhibit pancreatic beta-cell apoptosis (programmed cell death) and stimulate the proliferation and differentiation of insulin-secreting beta cells. In addition, GLP-1 inhibits gastric secretion and motility, which delay nutrient absorption and lead to less hunger. However, once in circulation, GLP-1 is quickly degraded by the enzyme dipeptidyl peptidase-4 (DPP-4).

GLP-1 agonists are pharmaceutical peptides (an injectable drug) that bind to GLP-1 receptors and express effects similar to that of GLP-1. Exenatide (Byetta®) was the first GLP-1 analog, introduced in April 2005. It was discovered as Exendin-4, a protein naturally secreted in the saliva and concentrated in the tail of the Gila monster. Exendin-4 shares extensive homology and function with mammalian GLP-1, but it has a therapeutic advantage because it resists degradation by DPP-4, which results in it staying active longer in the blood.

Liraglutide (Victoza®) is another GLP-1 agonist suitable for once-daily administration, but there are some warnings about liraglutide from rxlist.com:

> *Liraglutide causes dose-dependent and treatment-duration-dependent thyroid C-cell tumors at clinically relevant exposures in both genders of rats and mice. It is unknown whether Victoza® causes thyroid C-cell tumors, including medullary thyroid carcinoma (MTC), in humans, as human relevance could not be ruled out by clinical or nonclinical studies.*

This is just one of many examples that illustrates the physician's task of determining the risk-benefit ratio when the risks are unknown. Both exenatide and liraglutide assist in weight reduction and do not cause hypoglycemia by themselves. The glucose-lowering potential of GLP-1 agonists is high in those who consume carbohydrates, but limiting side effects include nausea and vomiting, particularly early in the course of treatment.

Concerns regarding an increased risk of pancreatitis remain unresolved. The cost of these drugs is high compared with metformin and sulfonylureas. These drugs have potential value for those following a ketogenic diet as they assist in fat loss, do not cause hypoglycemia by themselves, and have been reported to help suppress carbohydrate cravings.[87]

Dipeptidyl Peptidase-4 (DPP-4) Inhibitors

As mentioned in the previous section, dipeptidyl peptidase-4 (DPP-4) is an enzyme that degrades and inactivates GLP-1. By inhibiting this enzyme, the effect and duration of naturally produced GLP-1 can be amplified. The oral drugs in this class include sitagliptin (Januvia), vildagliptin (Galvus), saxagliptin (Onglyza), linagliptin (Tradjenta) and alogliptin, anagliptin, and teneligliptin in Japan.

The first agent in this class to come to market was sitagliptin, approved by the FDA in 2006. Although the glucose-lowering potential is modest (expected HbA1c reduction: 0.5%–1.0%), the drugs in this class are generally well tolerated, are weight neutral, and do not cause hypoglycemia by themselves. The cost of these drugs is high compared with metformin and sulfonylureas. There is some concern about pancreatitis in the use of these drugs, as discussed in a perspective review by a team from Aristotle University in Greece.[88]

α-Glucosidase Inhibitors

The oral drugs in this class include acarbose, miglitol and voglibose. They are not systemically absorbed and work by delaying absorption of carbohydrates from the intestine. They are used infrequently in the United States and Europe, and they are not known to cause hypoglycemia by themselves. This class of drug improves postprandial glucose excursions in those who consume carbohydrates. Their glucose-lowering potential is modest (expected HbA1c reduction: 0.5%–1.0%) in those who consume carbohydrates, and they are associated with gastrointestinal side effects, including flatulence and diarrhea. Because the mechanism of action is delay of carbohydrate absorption, this class of medication would not be expected to be effective while on a ketogenic diet.

Amylin Mimetic

Currently, the only available amylin mimetic is SYMLIN® (pramlintide acetate), an injectable antihyperglycemic drug for use in individuals with T1DM or T2DM treated with insulin. Pramlintide is a synthetic analog of human amylin. Amylin is a naturally occurring neuroendocrine hormone that contributes to glucose control after meals. It works by three different mechanisms, only one of which is helpful to those following a ketogenic diet. First, amylin, as well as pramlintide, suppresses glucagon secretion by the pancreatic alpha cells. This helps lower blood glucose and HbA1c, however, it lowers glucose in a glucose-independent fashion and, therefore, can cause hypoglycemia. The other two mechanisms of action include slowing of carbohydrate absorption and suppressing appetite, both of which are afforded by a ketogenic diet.

In a meta-analysis of three studies done by Lee et al. and published in the *Annals of Family Medicine*, pramlintide (Symlin) was somewhat more effective than the placebo in T1DM patients using conventional insulin therapy, with a between-group difference in HbA1c levels of 0.2% to 0.3% (two studies), but it was no more effective than the placebo in one study. Pramlintide-treated patients with both T1DM and T2DM experienced more weight loss compared with placebo-treated patients, who tended to gain weight. Patients treated with pramlintide experienced more frequent nausea and severe hypoglycemia compared with patients treated with the placebo.[89] The glucose-lowering effectiveness of SYMLIN in those who consume carbohydrates is modest (expected HbA1c reduction: 0.5%–1.0%). The cost is high compared with metformin and sulfonylureas, and it would not be expected to add much benefit to the combination of a ketogenic diet, exercise and insulin.

Sodium-Glucose Cotransporter 2 (SGLT2) Inhibitors

SGLT2 inhibitors are the newest class of hypoglycemic agents for T2DM. Canagliflozin was approved by the FDA in 2013 and dapagliflozin in 2014. Ipragliflozin is the first SGLT2 inhibitor approved in Japan. Empagliflozin has recently been approved in Europe and the United States. These medications block the kidneys' ability to reabsorb filtered glucose, resulting in glucose appearing in the urine (glycosuria)—a situation that usually only occurs in persons with uncontrolled diabetes. The glucose-lowering effectiveness of SGLT2 inhibitors in those who consume carbohydrates is modest (expected HbA1c reduction: 0.5%–1.0%).

Full-dose SGLT2 inhibition induces a rapid increase in urinary-glucose excretion, ranging from 50 to 100 g/day, equally in men and women and lasting slightly longer than twenty-four hours. When on a ketogenic diet, this meets or exceeds the total daily-carbohydrate intake. Any glucose excreted in excess of the daily-carbohydrate intake must come from liver glycogenolysis and gluconeogenesis. This could place an unnecessary demand on the liver to produce glucose. That said, in persons with T2DM who are very insulin resistant, the major abnormality causing hyperglycemia is excess production of glucose by the liver.

Side effects of this drug include urinary tract infections, osmotic diuresis (similar effect to a diuretic), genital mycotic infections, euglycemic and hyperglycemic diabetic ketoacidosis, and hyperkalemia (high blood potassium), especially in persons with impaired kidney function. In addition, there has been concern raised in the use of SGLT2 inhibitors in insulin-requiring diabetes, in both T2DM and, particularly so, in T1DM, that they may increase the risk of euglycemic (blood glucose not particularly elevated) diabetic ketoacidosis.[90]

The fact that the blood glucose is not unusually elevated would tend to make both patients and their doctors not suspect the diagnosis of DKA. Correspondence published in the *Lancet* stated that

> *investigators of at least one study have reported an increased incidence of ketonuria among patients with type 1 diabetes treated with an SGLT inhibitor. Additionally, SGLT inhibition has been associated with increased glucagon concentration in patients with type 2 diabetes. Although insulinopenia is implicated indirectly in ketogenesis, glucagon is implicated directly and is potently lipolytic and ketogenic.*[91]

It is theoretically possible that a ketogenic diet could further increase the likelihood of that occurring, especially in those who require insulin therapy. For this reason, in our opinion, SGLT2 inhibitors should be used with extra caution or avoided altogether on a ketogenic diet.

Multiple Non-Insulin Hypoglycemic Drug Combinations

If glycemic control has still not been achieved after lifestyle changes and titration of metformin to the maximum tolerable dose, then one or more additional antidiabetic drugs are recommended. Drug recommendations depend on individual-specific factors as well as the mechanism of action, potential for weight gain, possible side effects, cost, risk of hypoglycemia, and glucose-lowering potential, as discussed in the previous sections. Thus, the decision must be customized to the patient, and this is a matter that must be decided between the patients and their physicians. A paper by Zintzaras et al. discusses drug combinations in T2DM drug treatments.[92]

10

Insulin and T2DM

Humans cannot live without insulin. For a minority of long-term T2DM patients who produce inadequate amounts of insulin, exogenous insulin therapy may be necessary if lifestyle changes and other antidiabetic medications fail to reduce blood sugars.

In previous sections, we have discussed the presence of insulin resistance in T2DM. The body responds to this situation by making more insulin (hyperinsulinemia) in an attempt to overcome the resistance.

Many of the associated adverse medical conditions associated with T2DM are a result of hyperinsulinemia, even before any elevations in blood sugar occur. Thus, it is important to take full advantage of the ketogenic diet to lower insulin resistance and lose excess body-fat, and to use the insulin-sensitizing effects of exercise and the medications reviewed in the previous chapter before considering the use of insulin.

If endogenous insulin levels are still low due to beta-cell exhaustion, treating T2DM with exogenous insulin after insulin resistance has been minimized is appropriate. However, treating T2DM with insulin while insulin resistance is unchecked can further increase the risk of associated medical conditions, such as heart disease, cancer, stroke, and vascular disease. Taking insulin in this situation would only be appropriate if all other therapies failed.

For those of you reading this book who do utilize insulin as a treatment method, in this chapter, we will discuss the specific details of utilizing insulin to manage T2DM. Please note that you should not change your insulin therapy without consulting with your doctor.

Insulin: Action, Peak and Duration

For all practical purposes, the primary differences between various insulin preparations are the onset of action, time to peak action, and the duration of action.

- *Onset of action* is the length of time it takes for insulin to reach your bloodstream and begin to lower blood glucose.
- *Time to peak action* is the time when insulin is at its "peak" or maximum effectiveness at lowering blood glucose.
- *Duration of action* is the length of time insulin continues to lower blood glucose.

This is important to understand because by using more than one type of insulin by injection, a fairly close match to normal human insulin secretion can be accomplished.

The terms *basal insulin* and *bolus insulin* refer to their functions in the treatment of insulin-requiring diabetes. The role of basal insulin, also known as background insulin, is to keep blood-glucose levels at consistent levels during periods between meals. Bolus insulin is a dose specifically taken at mealtimes to keep blood-glucose levels under control following a meal.

When treating insulin-requiring diabetes (either T1DM or T2DM) with exogenous (injected) insulin, the goal is to mimic the natural insulin-secreting pattern of the pancreas. Since pancreatic insulin is secreted on a minute-to-minute basis, and exogenous insulin is injected into subcutaneous fat, the two cannot be identical in effect. However, with the use of insulin analogs, endogenous insulin effects can be approximated with exogenous insulin.

⟩ Long-acting insulin analogs, such as detemir (Levemir), glargine (Lantus), Tresiba (degludec U200), and Toujeo (glargine U300), mimic basal pancreatic insulin secretion.

⟩ Rapid-acting lispro (Humalog), aspart (Novolog), and glulisine (Apidra) and short-acting regular insulin (Humulin Regular and

Novulin Regular) mimic bolus pancreatic insulin secretion that occurs during and after meals. Rapid-acting insulins begin to lower blood glucose about fifteen minutes after injection. The peak of action occurs one to two hours after injection, and they continue to work up to four to five hours. These time frames can vary from one person to another, and blood-glucose testing can be used to determine one's actual duration of action of rapid-acting insulin. Rapid-acting insulin should be injected before a meal if blood glucose is normal or high, or after the meal if blood glucose is low. It's important to postpone injecting a rapid-acting insulin until the meal is available and ready to eat. In other words, don't inject insulin on the promise of a meal coming, wait until it actually arrives. This will help avoid hypoglycemia.

> Short-acting insulin reaches your bloodstream usually within thirty minutes after injection. It peaks in the two to three-hour range and stays effective for three to six hours.

In addition, rapid-acting mealtime insulin is used as the bolus insulin for most individuals who have normal stomach (gastric) emptying time and, therefore, a normal rate of nutrient absorption. For those with delayed gastric emptying from diabetic gastroparesis, short-acting regular insulin is used as the bolus insulin since it will prevent postprandial hypoglycemia from the mismatch between rapid insulin absorption and the delayed nutrient absorption caused by diabetic gastroparesis.

We've provided a table that compares different insulin preparations as a reference. You can access it from the bottom of the "About this Site/Resources" page of the ketogenic-diet-resource.com website). Information presented in the table has been adapted from a document found online at camdenhealth.org.[93]

Consult with your physician to see if the instructions in the table might be right for you. Again, we strongly advise you to consult with your physician before you begin to make changes in the manner in which you take insulin, especially if you also begin the ketogenic diet at the same time.

NPH Insulin

NPH insulin (Humulin N, Novolin N, Novolin NPH, NPH Iletin II, and isophane insulin) has three potential problems compared to the newer basal-insulin analogs.

First, the protamine that is added to human insulin to make NPH can cause major life-threatening allergic reactions in some individuals if they receive protamine to reverse the effects of heparin (an antico-agulant) after various medical procedures.[94]

Second, because NPH insulin has a peak of action in the middle of the night when it is injected as long-acting insulin at dinnertime or bedtime, it can cause nighttime hypoglycemia more often than the long-acting basal insulin analogs.[95]

And third, NPH has an inconsistent absorption rate when injected subcutaneously, which makes glycemic control less predictable. There are many reasons for the variability of absorption rate; however, an important reason is that NPH is a suspended crystalline insulin rather than a soluble insulin.

Premixed insulin preparations contain both NPH and either regular or rapid-acting insulin in different fixed ratios. Mixing NPH with other insulins affects the bioavailability and variability of biphasic-insulin mixtures. More importantly, to get optimal blood-glucose control, patients need flexibility in choosing the correct basal and bolus insulin doses rather than having a fixed basal-to-bolus ratio. The analog basal insulins, glargine (Lantus), detemir (Levemir), Tresiba (degludec U200), and Toujeo (glargine U300), lack the abovementioned potential problems, but note that they cannot be mixed with any other insulins and, thus, require separate injections.

We refer you to a review article titled "Bioavailability and variability of biphasic insulin mixtures" by Søeborg et al. for a detailed discussion of other reasons for the variable degree of absorption and variable absorption rate of NPH insulin and NPH insulin mixtures.[96]

Carbohydrate Counting Doesn't Work

Both T1DM and T2DM individuals are taught to count carbohydrates while consuming a diet containing 45%–65% of energy from carbohydrates, particularly if they are taking insulin, trying to address hypoglycemic episodes, or trying to improve poor glycemic control. Most individuals find that this strategy is not very effective in achieving any of these goals and often blame themselves for their lack of success. It turns out that this self-blame is misplaced, as there are logical reasons for this lack of success.

The carbohydrate-counting method is based on a linear model. Using this linear model, each individual is supposed to determine how many units of insulin to inject for the number of grams of carbohydrate consumed. For example, you might initially determine that you need 1 unit of insulin for 20 grams of dietary carbohydrate. So, if your meal contains 80 grams of dietary carbohydrate, then you take 4 units of insulin. A study done by Marran et al. and published in *The South African Medical Journal* showed that this simple linear calculation is not based in reality.[97]

Using the linear carbohydrate-to-insulin ratio (carbohydrate counting) currently recommended by ADA and AACE, the study showed an exponential increase in after-meal blood-glucose excursions with increasing carbohydrate loads. Reasons for this exponential increase center on three variables:

1. Counting carbohydrate grams does not account for great variation in the actual amount of glucose absorbed from various carbohydrate-containing foods.

2. There is variation in the amount of insulin that gets absorbed from an injection site.

3. If protein content varies from meal to meal, it could throw off the results.

The combination of these variables largely explains why carbohydrate counting on a standard high-carbohydrate diet does not work for estimating insulin dosage. This may also help explain why choosing foods based on glycemic load while eating a higher-carb diet is not effective in achieving normal glycemic control. Several other studies have confirmed that the linear carbohydrate-to-insulin-ratio method is ineffective.

A meta-analysis of studies published in the *Lancet*, titled "Efficacy of carbohydrate counting in type 1 diabetes," examined the effectiveness of carbohydrate counting in T1DM and reported: "We identified seven eligible trials, of 311 potentially relevant studies, comprising 599 adults and 104 children with type 1 diabetes. Study quality score averaged 7.6 out of 13. Overall there was no significant improvement in HbA1c concentration with carbohydrate counting versus the control or usual care."[98]

A randomized controlled trial of 281 patients with type 2 diabetes done by Bergenstal et al. was designed to test the effect of carbohydrate counting on HbA1c compared to a standard insulin adjustment algorithm. The authors found there was no significant difference in HbA1c between the simple algorithm versus carb counting.[99]

In the GIOCAR study by Laurenzi et al., 56 persons with T1DM using an insulin pump were followed. One group of 26 were assigned to carbohydrate counting, while 26 controls continued their usual management. At twenty-four weeks, the intention-to-treat group, showed no significant difference between their HbA1c, hypoglycemic and hyperglycemic episodes and fasting blood-glucose values.[100]

The evidence shows that counting carbohydrates while on a high-carbohydrate diet is not an effective method for good glycemic control. The better solution is to reduce total carbohydrate intake to minimize blood-sugar excursions.

Insulin-Injection Techniques

Even though insulin doses will be lower while on the ketogenic diet, it's a good idea to rotate injections to different locations within your chosen body area to avoid the possibility of fat hypertrophy, a lump under the skin caused by accumulation of extra fat at the site of many subcutaneous injections of insulin. Below are some helpful injection techniques to follow:

> The areas chosen for injection should have some subcutaneous fat. Pinching up the skin before injecting can prevent the insulin from going into muscle if there isn't much subcutaneous fat. Injecting into muscle will accelerate the rate of insulin absorption and would typically be desirable only for treating high blood sugar with rapid-acting insulin. If you can't pinch up some skin, avoid that area, because there is not enough fat in that location.

> Using a shorter needle (6 mm) will also help prevent injecting into muscle.

> Skin should be cleaned, but alcohol swabs are not necessary.

> To minimize discomfort, insert the needle quickly. Slow insertion of the needle is more painful than rapid insertion.

> Sometimes a drop of blood will appear on the skin after removing the needle. Just apply mild pressure with a clean paper napkin, and it will stop bleeding in a few seconds. Should you get blood on your clothing, hydrogen peroxide will remove it.

> Sometimes a small amount of insulin will leak out of the injection site. The amount that leaks out is so small that it is unlikely to make much difference. Removing the needle more slowly after the injection can sometimes decrease or stop the leakage. Removing the needle slowly is not painful.

Insulin Pumps

Insulin pumps are an option for insulin-requiring diabetes. Insulin pumps are programmable devices that inject either rapid-acting or regular insulin into subcutaneous fat as a bolus for meals or to correct elevated blood sugar. They also provide a continuous infusion to mimic pancreatic basal-insulin secretion at an adjustable rate that is programmed by the user. Typically, rapid-acting insulin is used in order to more closely mimic pancreatic insulin secretion.

Because insulin doses are significantly smaller (typically half) on a ketogenic diet, it's important to choose an insulin pump that is able to deliver insulin at a rate compatible with your needs. For example, the OmniPod system can deliver insulin in increments of 0.05 units/hr while the smallest increment others deliver is 0.1 units/hr.

Other brands of insulin pumps include the One Touch Ping and MiniMed 530G. An insulin pump and real-time continuous glucose monitor can be used at the same time, but because the rt-CGMs are not accurate enough to be used to determine insulin therapy, this combination cannot be used as an artificial pancreas. On a side note, on September 28, 2016, the FDA approved the first hybrid closed loop system (artificial pancreas), the Medtronic's MiniMed 670G System, intended to automatically monitor blood sugar and adjust basal insulin doses in people with type 1 diabetes.

The MiniMed® 530G with Enlite® Sensor combines an insulin pump and rt-CGM, which communicates readings to the pump and can suspend the pump at a set low-glucose reading. It can also issue alerts for both low and high-glucose readings. This is an especially useful feature during sleep.

There are also potential complications related to insulin pump use. These include hyperglycemia, hypoglycemia, diabetic ketoacidosis related to pump or tubing malfunction, infection at the catheter site, and scar tissue at the insulin infusion site. It is advised that insulin pump users have insulin syringes and long-acting insulin available in the event of pump failure.

For some individuals, insulin pumps are advisable and can result in improved glycemic control with limited risk of adverse events. In a study by Johnson et al., which examined the long-term outcomes of insulin pump therapy in type 1 children, "a total of 345 patients on pump therapy were matched to controls on injections. The mean HbA1c reduction in the pump cohort was 0.6% (6.6 mmol/mol). This improved HbA1c remained significant throughout the 7 years of follow-up. Pump therapy reduced severe hypoglycemia from 14.7 to 7.2 events per 100 patient-years."[101]

Insulin Therapy for Type 2 Diabetes Mellitus

Due to the progressive pancreatic beta-cell dysfunction (most people maintain some endogenous insulin secretion even in the later stages of T2DM) that can occur with T2DM, insulin therapy sometimes becomes necessary to achieve adequate glucose control. If an individual cannot achieve glycemic control after exhausting other treatment avenues, such as a ketogenic diet, regular exercise, excess body-fat loss, and taking the maximum tolerable dose of antidiabetic drugs, then insulin is recommended.

Once glycemic control improves with the addition of insulin, one or more of the non-insulin hypoglycemic medications may be reduced or discontinued. The type and number of insulin injections depend on abnormalities in the glucose profile.

Basal-Insulin Therapy

Basal-insulin therapy is usually initiated in patients with T2DM who have elevated fasting blood glucose. It mimics the continuous pancreatic beta-cell secretion needed to facilitate glucose, protein and fat regulation between meals, during an overnight fast, and during prolonged fasting as might occur in unusual circumstances. This can also be accomplished with an insulin pump that uses a rapid-acting insulin such as lispro (Humalog), aspart (Novolog), glulisine (Apidra), or regular insulin. The injectable basal-insulin preparations are glargine (Lantus), detemir (Levemir), Tresiba (degludec U200), and Toujeo (glargine U300). They are usually started at a low dose and increased over time. Generally, Lantus is given once daily, but it can be given twice daily if that improves glycemic control. Levemir is approved for either once or twice daily, however, the pharmacodynamics of Levemir are different than Lantus, as shown in a study by Plank et al. The authors reported the following:

> Duration of action for insulin detemir was dose dependent and varied from 5.7, to 12.1, to 19.9, to 22.7, to 23.2 hrs for 0.1, 0.2, 0.4, 0.8, and 1.6 units/kg, respectively.[102]

This is important to understand because the duration of action decreases as the Levemir dose decreases as a result of the ketogenic diet. Therefore, a person on a ketogenic diet may find that the effect of once-daily Levemir wears off before 24 hours. For example, if a 150-pound person (68 kg) takes 14 units of Levemir once daily, the duration of action according to this study would be 12.1 hours (14 units/68 kg = 0.2 units/kg Levemir). The effect of Levemir would wear off 12 hours sooner than expected and would likely result in an increase in blood glucose. Giving Levemir twice daily would prevent this increase in blood glucose. Both Tresiba (degludec U200) and Toujeo (glargine U300) have longer durations of action and are given once daily.

Whether you give the evening basal-insulin dose at dinner or bedtime is determined by glycemic control during the night and in the morning. Some persons with a significant rise in blood sugar in the early morning hours (dawn phenomenon) find a bedtime dose more effective in suppressing early-morning hepatic-glucose production due to the normal early-morning rise in cortisol and growth hormone compared to a dinnertime dose. Similarly, some may find a bedtime dose more effective in preventing nighttime hypoglycemia compared to a dinnertime dose.

Most individuals can be taught to titrate their own insulin dose. The basal-insulin dose can be adjusted up or down by 1 to 2 units no more frequently than once or twice a week due to the long half-life of basal insulin. The dose of both Tresiba (degludec U200) and Toujeo (glargine U300) should be adjusted no more frequently than once a week. Of course, the basal-insulin dose must be decreased more frequently than the previous guidelines if nighttime or morning (fasting) hypoglycemia develops.

A correct basal-insulin dose allows a meal to be skipped if needed without resulting in either hypoglycemia or hyperglycemia. For those on an insulin pump, the basal-insulin rate serves the purpose of a basal-insulin injection and provides more flexibility in adjustment when conditions such as the level of exercise change. This is one advantage of insulin-pump therapy.

Mealtime Insulin Therapy

If fasting blood glucose is close to your target, but either the average blood glucose or HbA1c remains above your target blood-glucose goal and the one to two-hour postprandial blood glucose is consistently greater than 140–180 mg/dL despite several non-insulin hypoglycemic medications, then mealtime insulin with a rapid-acting or regular insulin may be necessary.

Even on a ketogenic diet, the protein and small amount of carbohydrate in a meal requires that insulin be available to metabolize the food and maintain normal blood sugars. It may be tempting to skip the mealtime insulin dose due to its much smaller size; however, this can result in several hours of elevated blood glucose after each meal. This can be avoided with small mealtime insulin doses and appropriate basal-insulin doses. Of course, there may be times when not taking mealtime insulin on a ketogenic diet is appropriate, for example, if one has low blood glucose before a meal and plans to exercise shortly afterward or finished exercising earlier.

A check of blood glucose before each meal is used to determine the correct dose of rapid-acting or regular mealtime insulin (or "bolus" with an insulin pump). The dose of mealtime insulin on a ketogenic diet will generally be significantly lower than when one is on a high-carbohydrate diet. Your doctor will likely advise you to start with a low dose, say 1 to 2 units for average sized adults (more for large or insulin resistant adults), and then adjust up or down over time. The total insulin dose chosen before meals is the insulin needed for the meal itself, plus or minus a corrective insulin dose, if any.

For example, if your target blood glucose is 96 mg/dL and your pre-meal blood glucose is 149 mg/dL, then you will need a larger mealtime insulin dose. If your rapid-acting insulin dose for dinner is 3 units, and you have estimated that a corrective dose factor of rapid-acting insulin will lower your blood glucose 30 mg/dL per unit of insulin, then your mealtime insulin dose will be 3 + (149 − 96)/30 = 4.75 units.

Similarly, if your pre-meal blood glucose is 73 mg/dL, then you will need a smaller mealtime insulin dose. In this example, you calculate 3 + (73 − 96)/30 = 2.25 units. It's prudent to err on the side of less insulin in cases where blood glucose is already low. In this example, the mealtime insulin dose would be 2 units. Note that this calculation assumes a constant linear relationship between insulin administered and the resulting blood glucose, which is not necessarily the case. It is an approximation at best. You can always give a correction insulin dose a few hours after the meal, if needed, but avoiding hypoglycemia is the highest priority.

The correction dose factor of 30 mg/dL per unit of insulin in the above example is not necessarily a constant. It can vary with time of day, insulin sensitivity related to current levels of exercise, changes in body weight, and the current level of blood glucose, which is nonlinear. Therefore, you should reassess the correction factor frequently.

An example of nonlinear glucose lowering is seen when 1 unit of rapid-acting insulin lowers blood glucose from 120 to 90 mg/dL (a reduction of 30 mg/dL), but the same dose only lowers it from 200 to 180 mg/dL (a reduction of 20 mg/dL). The cause of this nonlinear behavior of injected insulin is not known. However, keeping a written log of blood glucose, and noting the effect of corrective doses of insulin at times when food is not being consumed, can help determine your current correction factor.

Short-acting regular insulin (Humulin Regular and Novulin Regular), having a slower onset and peak action, is often used as mealtime insulin instead of rapid-acting insulin to prevent hypoglycemia for those with diabetic gastroparesis (delayed stomach emptying due to autonomic neuropathy). This is due to the fact that rapid-acting insulin can have its effect in lowering blood glucose faster than the protein and carbohydrate in a ketogenic meal can raise blood glucose. After a meal, it is important to have blood glucose return to your target level at the time when mealtime insulin has been completely absorbed. For rapid-acting insulin, this absorption time can vary from two to five hours, depending on the person, site of injection, dose injected, and timing of exercise.

Determining Duration of Insulin Action

As with many aspects of having and managing diabetes, there are many variables that are not necessarily predictable, and the duration of action of insulin is one of those variables. The best method to help determine the duration of action of your mealtime insulin is to simply measure your blood glucose every 30 minutes beginning 1.5 hours after injection, until blood glucose remains relatively constant.

The time after injection when blood glucose levels off is your duration of action for that type of insulin at that time of day, at your current body weight, present level of physical activity, and number of grams of carbohydrate and protein consumed. You can see that many aspects of *Diabetes Care* are contextual. Over time, the factors influencing blood glucose will be become more and more apparent by simply measuring your blood glucose and taking note of the contextual factors such as weight, exercise and diet.

T2DM Insulin Management Skills: An Example

We will use Jim as an example patient to illustrate several diabetes-management skills. Jim has been a normal weight T2DM patient (80 kg = 176 lbs) for the past twenty-five years. He chooses to eat two meals a day, breakfast and dinner, because he's busy at work and never seems to be hungry on his ketogenic diet. He takes metformin 1,000 mg twice daily, Januvia 50 mg daily (down from 100 mg due to the recent addition of Lantus to avoid hypoglycemia). Two months ago, he was started on Lantus 15 ± units (divided into two injections) at bedtime due to persistent elevation of fasting blood glucose. In the past several weeks, he has been taking 15 units of Lantus, and he knows he can change his dose based on his morning fasting blood-glucose readings. Last week, his doctor prescribed Humalog at mealtime, due to persistent postprandial hyperglycemia (>140 mg/dL), and stopped the Januvia to prevent hypoglycemia. It wasn't needed with intensive insulin therapy.

Jim wants to determine his mealtime insulin (Humalog) duration of action so he will know when to check his blood glucose after his Humalog injection. He measures his fasting blood glucose before breakfast at 96 mg/dL and eats his usual breakfast containing 15 grams of total carbohydrate from olives and an ounce each of Brazil nuts, macadamia nuts and pumpkin seeds. He gets a total of 55 grams of protein by including an additional 6 ounces of salmon and rounds out his fat intake by drinking unsweetened coffee with 2 tablespoons of coconut oil.

At 1.5 hours after injection of 2 units of Humalog, his blood glucose is 132 mg/dL; at 2 hours after injection his blood glucose is 113 mg/dL; at 2.5 hours after injection his blood glucose is 93 mg/dL; at three hours after injection his blood glucose is 95 mg/dL. Seeing that his blood glucose has leveled off, he concludes that the duration of action of Humalog is 2.5 hours. He now knows that 2.5 hours after each Humalog injection at breakfast, he should check his blood glucose. If his basal-insulin dose is correct or if he were not taking any basal insulin, then his next pre-meal blood glucose should remain constant. This duration of action test could be repeated after dinner the following day as well. Should his weight, insulin requirement, exercise regimen, body site of insulin injections, or protein or carbohydrate composition of breakfast change significantly, then repeating the test may be necessary.

Since there are so many variables involved in managing diabetes, keeping as many of them as constant as possible will help you achieve your target blood glucose. One of the variables pertinent to mealtime insulin is diet. Keeping protein and carbohydrate contents constant (and the carb content low, of course) at each meal will help you achieve your target blood glucose. Taking about 20 to 30 grams of protein at each meal or evenly dividing daily protein intake between each meal also helps maintain lean muscle mass as discussed in a commentary article from Dr. Donald Layman, an expert on protein metabolism.[103]

Now let's return to our T2DM patient, Jim, and go through a day of insulin and glucose management while eating a ketogenic diet. After two months of Lantus, he notes his fasting blood glucose is 96 mg/dL and blood-ketone level is 1.5 mM, both of which are right on target. He has his usual salmon, olives, nuts and seeds for breakfast. Before starting Humalog, his average post-breakfast blood glucose was 187 mg/dL. As with any new insulin dose decision, he starts low and adjusts later doses based on previous responses. This is why keeping a record of all blood-glucose readings and insulin doses is important, and Jim is glad he does that.

Jim decides to take 2 units of Humalog by injection. Now, 2.5 hours after breakfast, his blood glucose is 132 mg/dL. Assuming his basal-insulin dose is correct and he does nothing additional (e.g., exercise), his blood glucose would remain about the same at 132 mg/dL until the next meal. Since he chooses to eat two meals a day, his blood glucose would remain elevated for about 11 hours until dinner. Instead, he decides to take a corrective dose of rapid-acting insulin.

Jim calculates that his blood glucose is elevated by 132 – 96 = 36 mg/dL and decides to take 1 unit of Humalog. His blood glucose 2.5 hours later is 88 mg/dL, close enough to his target of 96 mg/dL. Now he can use this to calculate that 1 unit of Humalog lowers his blood glucose by 132 – 88 = 44 mg/dL. He makes note of this correction factor, but he knows that this could change in the future due to a change in weight, exercise, stress, or medications—and, sometimes, for unexplained reasons. Most people who have had diabetes for some time know that things keep changing. Managing diabetes well means being alert to changes so that an appropriate response can be made.

Jim finishes work at 4:00 pm and meets a friend at the gym for a game of racquetball. He checks his blood glucose before the game: it's 93 mg/dL. Jim plays an intense game with quite a few sprints for the ball. He feels fine but checks his blood glucose because he is driving home: it's 148 mg/dL. He concludes that the hormones released during exercise caused the increase in blood glucose, but his drive home is short so he does not take any insulin. By the time he gets home, it's 6:30 pm—time for dinner. Jim's pre-meal blood glucose is 140 mg/dL. He tries to keep his dinner carbohydrates and protein about the same each night. For dinner, he's planning to have a 6-ounce grilled beef patty with 2 tablespoons of Worcestershire sauce. He has a dinner plate full of non-starchy cooked vegetables (broccoli, Bok Choy, collard greens) with 2 tablespoons of butter. For dessert, he has 1 ounce each of macadamia nuts and pumpkin seeds, and unsweetened coffee with 3 tablespoons of heavy whipping cream.

He estimates that due to the extra grams of carbohydrates in the non-starchy vegetables at dinner, his Humalog dose should be 3 units. He decides to add a correction dose due to his elevated blood glucose of 126 mg/dL. He uses his Humalog dose-correction factor of 44 mg/dL per unit insulin as follows: (140 – 96)/44 = 1 unit Humalog, and, thus, he takes 3 + 1 = 4 units of insulin at the start of dinner. His dinner macronutrient totals are 25 grams of total carbohydrate from his non-starchy vegetables, Brazil and macadamia nuts, and 50 grams of protein, primarily from his 6-ounce beef patty and nuts. His daily totals come to 118 grams protein (or 1.5 grams/kg body weight), 40 grams total carbohydrate, and 190 grams fat. His macronutrient calorie ratios are 20% protein, 7% carbohydrate, 73% fat. He's keenly aware that the grams of protein and carbohydrate consumed are what's most important to track because they have a greater effect on blood sugar.

Jim normally does not track his intake this closely, however, knowing the nutritional composition of his diet can certainly be helpful if he has to diagnose a problem with high blood sugar or weight gain. Jim is also not concerned about the amount of saturated fat (SFA) he eats for two reasons. First, he is in nutritional ketosis, and that means he's a prodigious fat burner. Saturated and monounsaturated fats are burned preferentially while in nutritional ketosis. In a study by Volek and Phinney et al., the authors demonstrated that subjects on a ketogenic diet had a larger drop in serum saturated-fat levels after twelve weeks on a ketogenic diet, despite consuming more than three times as much saturated fat compared to subjects on a low-fat diet.[104]

Second, Jim knows that 56 of the 190 grams of fat in his meals came from coconut oil, which is mostly saturated fat. In addition, coconut oil is a special fat that contains medium-chain triglycerides that are delivered straight to the liver and largely converted to ketones while in nutritional ketosis. It is not unusual that adding coconut oil to a ketogenic diet results in a significant increase in blood-ketone levels in 3 to 4 hours. Jim checks his blood glucose 2.5 hours after dinner and finds his reading is 65 mg/dL. Jim decides to take one glucose tablet containing 4 grams of pure glucose. Fifteen minutes later, he retests his blood glucose to check it before going to bed: it's 98 mg/dL. He takes some cheese or other protein-containing snack to prevent recurrence of hypoglycemia in light of his exercise. He's thrilled with his results but makes note of the possibility that his hypoglycemia was due to the 1 unit corrective dose of Humalog at dinner that he apparently did not need due to improved insulin sensitivity from his racquetball game in the afternoon. He also notes that this improved insulin sensitivity may last for an additional 24 to 48 hours after the exercise.[105, 106]

Jim records his exercise sessions, blood glucose, ketone levels, and insulin doses on his log to aid in his glycemic management.

The above scenario illustrates that management of diabetes may not be easy. It requires careful thought, record keeping, discipline with the ketogenic diet, and frequent blood-glucose and ketone monitoring. The good news is all of this can result in improved glycemic control and a reduction in hypoglycemic and hyperglycemic episodes. Jim can be certain that if he continues to carefully manage his diabetes, he will likely be free of long-term complications and escape the shortened lifespan typical of many people with diabetes.

Part 4

Exercise, Obesity, and Other Factors

11

The Role of Exercise

We believe exercise is an important part of a healthy lifestyle and that it plays an important role in health maintenance.[107] However, before starting any exercise program, consult with your physician. If you have coronary artery disease, known or unknown, starting an exercise program can precipitate a coronary event such as a heart attack or arrhythmia.

Once you have your doctor's clearance, an exercise program that gradually progresses in duration and intensity will be beneficial in the longer term. Even if you haven't exercised on a regular basis for years, it's not too late to start.

It is a common myth that the purpose of exercise is to burn calories to assist with weight loss. However, the data supporting this view is weak, and there are small, well-controlled studies that contradict this viewpoint.[108, 109] However, what is clear is that exercise improves insulin sensitivity, which is especially beneficial for persons with T2DM.[110, 111]

Exercise can improve many health markers, and it increases muscle insulin sensitivity, which translates to improved glycemic control and fewer diabetic medications and/or smaller insulin doses. Even for those who are sedentary, a single exercise session can improve glucose uptake in muscle. After a single session of moderate-intensity exercise, glucose uptake can increase by at least 40%. Many studies show that improvement in insulin sensitivity diminishes within sixteen to seventy-two hours after the last exercise session, so regular exercise is needed to maintain improved insulin sensitivity. Regular exercise also results in the development of other highly beneficial physical changes:

- Stronger bones, muscles, and tendons
- Stronger heart and lungs[112]
- Improved balance and resistance to falls
- Improved mental health

Although it's a popular reason, burning calories should not be a goal of exercise, even if you desire to lose excess body fat. Despite the appealing concept, practicing caloric balance is impossible. Given the varied factors involved, it's not possible to accurately track caloric intake or caloric expenditure. In addition, exercise does not burn as many calories as most people believe. You can spend sixty minutes walking and burn off 190 calories, then eat those same calories in the form of a doughnut in less than one minute.

We have heard too many people say "I exercise so I can eat what I want." Generally, that means so they can eat starches and sugary foods. Go to any large endurance sporting event and you are likely to see many overweight people finishing near the back of the pack. These overweight but fit people seem to contradict the idea that exercise assists in fat loss. We believe that their good intentions are thwarted by a high-carbohydrate diet and "carb loading" that is so popular in the sports world. They aren't aware that the effects of carbohydrate intake on blood sugar and insulin override the effects of exercise in the regulation of fat storage. It's clear that exercise cannot reverse the unhealthy effects of a poor diet, however, the addition of exercise to a ketogenic diet can do wonders for reversing insulin resistance and poor glycemic control. Exercise places demands on the circulatory system to increase blood flow, on the pulmonary system to increase blood oxygen, on the temperature regulatory system to cool the body, and on the metabolic system to provide nutrients to exercising muscles. It also enhances the effect of a ketogenic diet.

Carb-Adapted versus Keto-Adapted Muscles

Many people wonder how to fuel themselves with carbohydrates or other nutrients before, during, and after athletic training and events.

We believe the strategy should be different from the "carbohydrate loading" advice usually given.

For the past sixty years or so, athletes have been taught that muscles perform best with carbohydrates. Fat-adaptation has not been on their radar at all. These athletes have been taught to eat carbohydrates before, during, and after exercise. Eating carbohydrates just before exercise increases glycogen stores in both muscle and liver. Those carbohydrates also increase insulin secretion, which inhibits fat oxidation and ketone production.

Chronic carbohydrate ingestion also results in muscles that are carb-adapted and, therefore, dependent upon glucose and glycogen as energy sources. The majority of athletes are carb-adapted, so they must consume some form of carbohydrate to supply the glucose that their muscles require, especially during prolonged aerobic exercise. While this may not be a problem for young, lean, insulin-sensitive athletes, many others may store and retain excess fat or develop metabolic syndrome or diabetes as they get older, despite their exercise.

Athletes with a carbohydrate-fueling strategy can also run out of glycogen stores and "bonk" or "hit the wall." Because the carb-adapted athlete does not have the metabolic flexibility to burn fat at a sufficient rate, nor the ability to ingest enough carbohydrate to match energy expenditure, the supply of energy eventually fails to sustain athletic performance.

Dr. Jeff Volek showed that athletes who had been fat and keto-adapted by following a low-carbohydrate diet (LC) for months were able to utilize fat at a rate 2.3 times that of high-carb-adapted (HC) athletes. A new finding was that LC athletes had equal levels of muscle glycogen pre-exercise, immediately post-exercise, and two hours post-exercise as the HC athletes. Thus, moderate-intensity exercise can certainly be fueled with a low-carbohydrate diet. Although not formally studied in patients with diabetes, improved fat and ketone utilization by muscle during exercise certainly has potential advantages for those with diabetes, including less risk of hypoglycemia, particularly for those who take insulin, meglitinide, or sulfonylurea medications for diabetes.[113]

Exercise also leads to other improvements in well-being, as shown in many health markers, and so we encourage all those with diabetes to make the effort to incorporate a regular, enjoyable exercise routine into their lifestyle after they have been screened by their physicians to participate.

Benefits of a Ketogenic Diet for Diabetic Athletes

Becoming fat-adapted and keto-adapted can provide the diabetic athlete with several advantages. Being keto-adapted means that enzymes and transport proteins needed in every step of fat and ketone production and utilization are enhanced. Thus, the following factors are increased:

- Access to fat stores
- Ability to make ketones
- Ability to oxidize fatty acids and ketones for energy

Similarly, the body no longer needs as much muscle glycogen, which can decrease by as much as 50% in the fat-adapted athlete.[114] However, a more recent study of fat-adapted athletes by Jeff Volek showed that muscle-glycogen stores were not depleted and that less glycogen and more than twice as much fat was oxidized (burned) for muscle energy.[113] Thus, becoming fat-adapted means that muscles burn fatty acids and ketones preferentially and are less dependent on glucose.

In summary, becoming keto-adapted provides potential benefits to the diabetic athlete, including a reduction in hypoglycemia, hyperglycemia, and fuel exhaustion and improvement in fuel flow and energy utilization from readily accessible fat stores. Since there are factors that tend to both increase and decrease blood glucose during exercise, the blood-glucose response to exercise is not necessarily predictable. In those with T2DM who take insulin, sulfonylurea or meglitinide medications, be prepared to test blood glucose and treat, if needed, with glucose tablets or liquid before, during and after exercise. For those taking insulin, decreasing the dose of basal and/or rapid-acting insulin before exercise may also help prevent hypoglycemia.

Keto-Adaptation for Non-Diabetic Athletes

Are there advantages of becoming fat-adapted and keto-adapted for non-diabetic athletes? The possibility does indeed exist, and there are elite ultramarathon athletes winning and setting course records while on a low-carbohydrate diet. For example, Timothy Olsen is a low-carb athlete, and he is the current record holder of the 100-mile Western States Ultramarathon with a time of 14:46:44.[115] Zach Bitter, another low-carb athlete, has set several ultramarathon records, including the current 100-Mile American record with a time of 11:47:21.[116]

High-Intensity Interval Training

Whenever possible, get up and get moving! Any kind of exercise is great, but a type called high-intensity interval training (HIIT) may be the key to reducing insulin resistance. In a paper by Gibala et al., the authors wrote the following:

> *Arguably the best evidence to date regarding the potential for nutritional manipulation to enhance physiological adaptation to interval training is research on carbohydrate (CHO) restriction protocols. As originally proposed by Hansen et al. the basic concept is that training in a CHO-restricted state and/or with reduced glycogen availability could serve to augment the acute molecular signaling response to exercise... From a basic science standpoint, studies have shown that CHO-restricted training can enhance mitochondrial adaptation, even in highly trained individuals.*[117]

HIIT is exercise that is brief, infrequent and intense. It has different metabolic effects than lower-intensity exercise like long walks or distance running. Keep in mind that levels of exercise are individually driven. If a person is significantly overweight and out of shape, low-intensity exercise might be high-intensity exercise at first. Over time, as a person continues an exercise program, the gains in strength and agility will allow for an increase in exercise intensity.

Here are some examples of high-intensity exercise versus low-intensity exercise. Again, please get your doctor's approval before starting any exercise program.

Low-Intensity Exercise	High-Intensity Training
Walking or jogging slowly for a mile, five days a week.	Walk for five minutes to warm up. Then sprint as fast as you can for thirty seconds, then walk for four minutes to recover. Repeat this two to three more times, and do the whole routine only two times per week.
Riding a stationary bike at a medium speed for an hour, six days a week.	Ride a stationary bike at a medium speed for ten minutes, then pedal as fast as you can for thirty to sixty seconds, then slow down again to medium speed for four minutes. Repeat two to three times, and do this two times a week.
Lifting weights using light weights and lots of repetitions.	Use the heaviest weight you can lift safely, and lift it very slowly. For instance, you might do a leg press, take ten seconds to push the weight away, and then take ten seconds to bring it back. Do that again, four to five more times. The goal is to keep the muscle under a full weight load for the duration of the movement.

All of these high-intensity interval training methods have been used in various studies and protocols and have been shown to increase insulin sensitivity, improve fat loss and generally result in more retention of muscle mass and better fitness in a much shorter time than steady state, low-intensity exercise like walking. Some studies have shown that the effect of HIIT is more beneficial for men than women, and a small percentage of study participants have exhibited worse scores on a glucose tolerance test after HIIT training. In particular, Martin Gibala's team in the Department of Kinesiology at McMaster University in Ontario, Canada, has done some definitive research in this area. However, for those who are insulin resistant, HIIT does provide substantial benefits. In a 2014 paper, Dr. Gibala's team reports that

> subjects with insulin resistance have been reported to derive a greater training-induced change in glucose tolerance than age and BMI-matched normoglycemic controls, with men having larger improvements in insulin sensitivity than women.[118]

The bottom line is that exercise provides great benefits for people with diabetes, and we encourage everyone to start an exercise program if they don't already have one.

Aerobic Exercise Is Good Too

Although high-intensity exercise is a great way to increase fitness without spending hours at the gym, regular aerobic exercise, like brisk walking and slow jogging, has beneficial effects on blood-sugar control and insulin sensitivity as well. In fact, adding extra activity while going through your daily routine is beneficial. For instance, the following activities are easy to incorporate into your day, and, over time, they can make a significant difference in managing insulin sensitivity and achieving better blood-glucose levels.

- Walk to nearby destinations instead of driving
- Get off the bus a stop early and walk the rest of the way

- Work in the garden, rake leaves or wash the car
- Play actively with kids or pets
- Walk around while talking on the phone
- Park at the far end of store lots and walk
- Avoid elevators and escalators and choose to take the stairs as often as possible

A study published in the Global Journal of Health Sciences looked at a group of 53 diabetic women. Researchers had 27 women follow an exercise protocol 3 times a week for 8 weeks, while the remaining 26 acted as a control group and did not exercise. The exercise protocol included stretching and flexibility exercises for 10 minutes followed by walking for 30 minutes at medium intensity and then 10 more minutes of stretching. After 8 weeks, there were significant improvements in waist and hip circumference, insulin resistance, fasting glucose and plasma insulin for members of the group that exercised.[119] Another study by Cuff et al. showed that combining aerobic exercise with weight training had an even greater positive effect on insulin sensitivity for people with diabetes.[120]

12

Obesity, Diabetes, and Weight Loss

About 85% of persons with T2DM are overweight or obese. The metabolic changes that occur with both fat storage in adipose tissue and diabetes are similar, which explains their frequent coexistence. The common link between these conditions is insulin resistance. Experts say the cause of insulin resistance is unclear, but they insist that most likely it's caused by excess weight and physical inactivity. If you ask those same experts what causes excess weight gain, they will likely say, "eating too much and exercising too little." In other words, our body is like a barrel, if we pour too many calories in by eating too much, and don't drain them out by exercising too little, it will overflow, and we'll become obese. However, our bodies are much smarter than this simple equation suggests.

Fat-tissue storage and blood sugar are both carefully regulated by many hormones. These hormones include insulin, growth hormone, cortisol, glucagon, epinephrine, leptin, norepinephrine, testosterone, estrogen, and progesterone. Given that obesity and diabetes were unusual conditions in the past, the more likely explanation is one in which dietary changes play a role.

The carbohydrate hypothesis best explains numerous observations about the timing and food environment before and after the onset of obesity and diabetes. Even after thousands of years, diabetes and obesity were exceedingly rare in cultures living off the land. Only when a native diet of grass-fed meat, game, fish and eggs was changed by the influence of Western foods, rich in refined starches and sugar, did these problems erupt.

The transformation from health to obesity and diabetes in the Pima, an American Indian tribe, is a prime example. In the late 1800s, settlers on their route to the California gold rush passed through Pima territory in Arizona. They relied on the Pima for food and supplies. Many settled upstream, overtook the Pima's access to fish in the Gila River, and diverted the river's water flow to irrigate their crops, leaving little water for the Pima.

The Pima went from prosperous to poor in a span of forty years and became dependent on rations from the US government to avoid starvation. Half of the calories in the rations came from flour and sugar. Obesity in the Pima population soon became prevalent, and diabetes followed. Fast forward to 1979: a study by Knowler et al. reported that the Pima tribe had the highest prevalence of diabetes ever recorded: 21.1% of the population.[121]

Many claim that the Pima have a genetic predisposition for diabetes. Although that may be true, the environmental conditions must be present for the genetic susceptibility to become evident. Food in the United States, and now in most of the world, is composed primarily of processed foods high in refined starches and sugar.

This is likely the major cause of the current pandemic of obesity and T2DM. Removing these substances from our diet has the potential to improve glycemic control in both T1DM and T2DM, place T2DM in remission as long as pancreatic beta-cell insulin production is not yet severely impaired, and reverse the pandemic of obesity and T2DM throughout the world.

Will that happen? Perhaps, but there would have to be an acceptance of the carbohydrate hypothesis by governments of the major food-producing countries. The production of refined starches and sugars is very profitable, and food companies are not likely to voluntarily give up those profits.

The US government has been subsidizing starch and sugar-producing crops since 1922.[122] Direct-payment subsidies are provided without regard to the economic need of the recipients nor the financial condition of the farm economy. Established in 1996, direct payments were originally meant to wean farmers off traditional subsidies that are triggered during periods of low prices for corn, wheat, soybeans, cotton, rice, and other crops. From a public-health perspective, it is difficult to understand why the federal government subsidized tobacco farmers an average of $127 million per year until that subsidy ended in 2014. But this pales in comparison to the most heavily US-subsidized crop—corn!

The average yearly corn subsidy in the United States over the past seventeen years has been $4.97 billion. Corn is used heavily in numerous processed foods in the production of high-fructose corn syrup, and to feed animals that were never meant to eat corn. Feeding animals corn results in various unique illnesses and adversely affects body composition, making the food product less healthy for humans to consume. Corn is produced in such excess that it is used to produce ethanol as a gasoline supplement and substitute.

As we've discussed, a steady diet of processed foods made from refined starches and sugar elevates blood-insulin levels. Insulin controls the entry and exit of fat from adipose tissue, and elevated levels of insulin increase fat storage and block metabolic access to stored fat so that it can't be used to fuel the body. Over time, refined-carbohydrate consumption and the associated insulin response lead to insulin resistance. Insulin resistance leads to increased hepatic-glucose production and a decreased ability of numerous body cells to take up glucose, starting with muscle and then with the liver and adipose cells. Because adipose cells remain sensitive to insulin's message to store carbohydrate for a longer period of time than muscle and liver cells, they continue to store fat under the direction of increased circulating insulin.

There is no controversy regarding these mechanisms and the association of dietary refined-carbohydrate consumption to excess fat storage. Nevertheless, dietary recommendations to reduce carbohydrate intake, which should logically result from this evidence, are in conflict with the entrenched lipid-heart hypothesis that states that cholesterol and fat are the cause of our health problems.

USDA dietary guidelines are meant to apply to all Americans, but since the first publication of these guidelines in 1980[123], the prevalence of obesity and diabetes in the United States has tripled. Perhaps the recommendations could be customized to specific groups of individuals. Perhaps those who are overweight, obese, or diabetic could be told the truth:

- Refined carbohydrates and sugar cause obesity and T2DM

- Carbohydrates are unnecessary macronutrients

- People with T1DM and T2DM are intolerant of carbohydrates

- Dietary-fat consumption, other than processed vegetable oils and trans fats, does not lead to atherosclerosis, peripheral vascular disease, heart disease, or stroke *unless* accompanied by refined carbohydrates

If the American population knew the truth and stopped buying refined-carbohydrate products, the food industry would be forced to stop production of carbohydrate-based convenience foods and make healthier foods in order to stay in business. Then, as the marketplace changed, our current health pandemic might begin to reverse.

Why Ketogenic Diets Induce Weight Loss

Shedding excess body fat is never easy, particularly when weight-loss advice is "eat less, exercise more, and avoid dietary fat." For many who can stick to a dietary regimen but are insulin resistant and hyperinsulinemic, a calorie-restricted low-fat diet simply does not lower insulin levels enough, and it is energy and nutrient deficient. This combination leads to hunger. Dr. Robert C. Atkins put it this way:

The main reason low-calorie diets fail in the long run is because you go hungry on them … And while you may tolerate hunger for a short time, you can't tolerate hunger all your life.

The low-carbohydrate ketogenic diet addresses insulin resistance and hyperinsulinemia by restricting the very dietary components that cause it: refined carbohydrates and sugar. In contrast to the low-fat and calorie-restricted diet, the carbohydrate-restricted ketogenic diet effectively addresses obesity *without* caloric restriction for most people.

Remember, insulin resistance and hyperinsulinemia are equivalent to carbohydrate intolerance. The greater the carbohydrate intolerance, the more dietary carbohydrate restriction is needed to correct insulin resistance and hyperinsulinemia and, thus, to lose excess fat.

In advanced stages of insulin resistance, many people seeking a solution may have surpassed the point where the elimination of refined carbohydrates and sugar is enough to correct metabolic abnormalities. This is why a ketogenic diet also restricts foods that are high in all carbohydrates, even if they are not refined. These foods include potatoes and sugar-rich fruits, such as bananas, grapes, and mangos. You may not like the idea of restricting these foods entirely, but if you have severe insulin resistance, it may be your best solution for reversing this condition.

The majority of foods people crave contain insulin-stimulating carbohydrates and sugar. The insulin surge that occurs after a carbohydrate-predominant food is consumed sends a rewarding signal to the brain. This reward signal is then associated with that food. This has been observed in animals as well. By restricting these foods for several weeks, the strong desire to eat them fades.

Low-Fat, Calorie-Restricted Diet versus a Ketogenic Diet

Let's clarify the difference between a calorie-restricted, low-fat diet and the ketogenic diet. The difference is really a matter of fuel flow based on the effects of insulin. Insulin drives the storage and release of fat from adipose tissue. If insulin levels are elevated, the release of stored fat for fueling the body is blocked. Because a calorie-restricted, low-fat diet restricts all macronutrients but does not restrict carbohydrates enough to fully correct insulin resistance and high insulin levels, insufficient amounts of fat are released from adipose tissue to supply the body's energy needs. So, not only is fat unavailable to fuel the body, glucose intake is also insufficient because calories are restricted. The body is smart enough to recognize a fuel deficiency, even if scientists don't understand all the signals at play.

If a disciplined dieter on a calorie-restricted, low-fat diet resists hunger, either reactive hypoglycemia develops, forcing the person to seek out carbohydrate foods, or, if blood sugar remains close to normal, the body reduces or slows its metabolism to match the energy deficit it experiences. This is often why the overweight or obese person does not like to exercise: hyperinsulinemia is keeping energy stores tucked away in adipose tissue, and the body is conserving energy to compensate. The net result is unsustainable hunger, reactive hypoglycemia, and modest weight loss at best. Often, weight loss includes lean muscle loss due to an energy deficit in the presence of relative hyperinsulinemia.

In contrast, the ketogenic diet helps correct insulin resistance and hyperinsulinemia. In a metabolic setting of low insulin levels, adipose tissue readily gives up its fat stores in the form of fatty acids. Most of the body's tissues can readily use them for fuel. For the few tissues that cannot use fatty acids (brain, red blood cells, cornea, kidney medulla), the liver converts fatty acids to a fuel in the form of ketones and converts glycerol and leftover amino acids from protein to glucose. It is this abundance of available fuel that explains why calorie restriction is neither needed nor desired on a ketogenic diet. Essentially, the body is already consuming a high-calorie meal, only the calories are coming from the body's own fat stores. The person may, in fact, be consuming fewer calories in his or her diet, but the body is not aware of this because of the abundant amount of fat being released from adipose tissue. In other words, the body cannot distinguish between fatty acids coming from the diet versus adipose tissue as the source. All it knows is that its energy needs are being met. In summary:

> *Calorie-restricted diet* means the body is not getting enough calories to cover energy expenditures and satisfy hunger.

> *Calorie-unrestricted ketogenic diet* means the body is getting all the energy it needs from fat stores, even if the diet is not providing all of the calories needed.

A ketogenic diet used for weight loss may be lower in calories, but the resulting energy deficit is replaced with fat mobilized from adipose tissue. Once you understand the concept, you begin to wonder why anyone would recommend a calorie-restricted diet in the first place. Would they also recommend an energy-restricted diet or a vitamin-deficient diet?

Factors Affecting Weight Loss with a Ketogenic Diet

When T2DM develops in an obese person, we know that insulin resistance and hyperinsulinemia are present to a marked degree. The logical treatment of obesity and being overweight, especially in the setting of T2DM, is restriction of dietary refined carbohydrates and sugar, which are likely the causative agents in the first place. To overcome the greater magnitude of insulin resistance and hyperinsulinemia, not only do dietary refined carbohydrates and sugar need to be restricted, but total dietary-carbohydrate load needs to be restricted as well.

Persons with T2DM are generally intolerant of carbohydrates with the exception of a few carbs from non-starchy vegetables, nuts and seeds, and low-sugar fruits. Adding medications to control blood sugar, either by forcing the already impaired beta cells to secrete more insulin or by giving insulin injections, makes managing excess fat stores with T2DM a true challenge. It's not a challenge that can't be conquered, but it is a challenge all the same. A strict ketogenic diet will be needed, at least initially, with about 20 to 50 grams of total carbohydrates per day, depending on several factors, which include your degree of insulin resistance, the amount and regularity of exercise (due to its beneficial effect on insulin resistance), your degree of adiposity, and medications you may be taking.[124]

Once glycemic control and body fat improves to target, then cautiously adding back some carbohydrates in small increments may be feasible. However, do not let yourself add back too many carbohydrates. In addition to non-compliance with the ketogenic diet, this is the most common reason for deteriorating glycemic control and body-fat regain. If you no longer miss the carbohydrate-containing foods you used to eat, and you have reached your goal weight, additional fat can be added to the diet to maintain your goal weight. Following the steps mentioned above for implementing a ketogenic diet should result in weight loss for most with T2DM carrying extra weight.

Intermittent Fasting

Intermittent fasting simply means not snacking between meals, extending the time between meals, or eating fewer than three meals per day. Intermittent fasting can help reduce insulin resistance and hyperinsulinemia in those with glucose intolerance, prediabetes and T2DM. This can provide additional benefits when a ketogenic diet, excess bodyfat loss, exercise, and insulin-sensitizing medications are not enough to normalize insulin resistance and hyperinsulinemia.

If you need additional improvement in your blood-sugar levels after following the ketogenic diet carefully and strictly for several months, you can try reducing the number of meals eaten each day in order to reduce baseline blood-insulin levels. Keep in mind that intermittent fasting refers to the timing of eating, not the macronutrient or caloric intake. Macronutrient intake and caloric requirements are calculated as described in chapter 5, and reducing the number of meals per day may (or may not) involve eating somewhat larger meals.

The combination of a ketogenic diet and intermittent fasting with exercise, excess body-fat loss, and possibly insulin-sensitizing medications should be enough to markedly improve the most severe case of insulin resistance. Some people will choose to have two meals a day: lunch and dinner, for example. This way, there will be an 18-hour period of fasting each day. Also, every day doesn't have to be the same. You can have one meal three days a week and two meals four days a week, for example. You can devise your own schedule to fit your lifestyle. Since the ketogenic diet effectively reduces appetite, it facilitates intermittent fasting, and this strategy can help improve or resolve insulin resistance and improve blood sugars in those with T2DM.

Total Fasting

We do not recommend going beyond twenty-four hours without food for the treatment of diabetes. Doing so can result in loss of lean body mass (i.e., muscle). Most of the loss of muscle occurs in the first days of a prolonged fast. A study by Cahill et al. shows that the muscle losses are similar for both normal and diabetic subjects.[125] As the body begins to make ketones from fat to replace glucose that is derived from protein and to some extent from glycerol in fat, the rate of muscle loss decreases, but it never approaches zero. As detailed in Dr. George Cahill's 1973 lecture on ketosis,[126] the amount of muscle loss can be calculated by multiplying the grams of nitrogen lost in the urine by 22.7 to yield the number of grams of muscle/lean tissue lost each day.

By the end of the first day of fasting, the body will lose 0.65 pounds of muscle. After one week of fasting, the body is losing 0.5 pounds of muscle each day and a cumulative loss of 4 pounds. After two weeks of fasting, the body is losing 0.4 pounds of muscle each day and a cumulative loss of 7.3 pounds. After three weeks of fasting, the body is losing 0.3 pounds of muscle each day and a cumulative loss of 9.75 pounds. After 38 days of fasting, an obese, non-diabetic man is losing 0.25 pounds of muscle each day and a cumulative loss of 14 pounds. The danger in this loss is that a portion of that muscle loss is coming from your heart and can lead to serious problems, including heart failure, cardiac arrhythmias, and death.

There are quite a few documented deaths from prolonged fasting in the literature, which is why doctors stopped using them for severe obesity.[127]

Can some people go for several days, or even a few weeks, without eating and not die from it? Of course. In fact, there is one case report in the literature of a man who decided to extend a medically supervised fast beyond the recommended time for slightly more than a year. He was monitored by physicians and required some electrolyte and mineral supplementation, but nothing ominous occurred.[128] However, you can cross a street with a blindfold on and not be hit by a car, sometimes. But you probably wouldn't advise your family or friends to do that.

13

Other Factors to Consider

The following information is offered on common questions about the ketogenic diet.

Ketogenic Diet and Vegetarianism

Recommendations for treating diabetes with a ketogenic diet call for a carbohydrate intake of less than 50 grams per day, with the goal of reducing blood sugar and insulin levels. For most people, eating a moderate amount of protein and staying below an intake of 50 grams of carbohydrate per day results in ketosis.

Adhering to a vegetarian diet that restricts animal fats and proteins necessarily requires eating more carbohydrate. This higher carbohydrate intake can have the effect of increasing baseline blood sugar and short-circuiting ketosis. It is possible to eat a lower-carb vegetarian diet. A book called the *New Atkins for a New You: The Ultimate Diet for Shedding Weight and Feeling Great* by Dr. Eric Westman, Dr. Jeff Volek and Dr. Stephen Phinney is recommended as it has a vegetarian section, as does the Atkins website.

As stated on the Atkins website, the recommendation for carbohydrate intake for vegetarians start at 30 carbohydrates per day, which is right in line with a ketogenic diet for diabetes. Those who follow a variation of a vegetarian diet will discover that eggs, dairy, and fish are excellent sources of protein, fat and many micronutrients. A vegan diet, which excludes all animal products, is more challenging because legumes and soy become major sources of protein. These protein sources also contain significant amounts of carbohydrate that can prevent ketosis. Nevertheless, a carbohydrate-restricted vegan diet would be more beneficial than the Standard American Diet for those with diabetes. Googling vegetarian or vegan low-carb diet will identify resources on the web that might help.

How Long Should I Stay on the Diet?

A change to better eating habits should be permanent so that the resulting benefits are also permanent. Going back to your old high-carb eating habits will only result in a loss of blood-sugar control, blood-sugar elevations and diabetic complications, and you'll be right back where you started. Rather than a temporary change, think of this diet as a new way of eating that helps you regain your health and your life.

How Stress Affects Ketosis

Stress can be a confounding factor for achieving your target blood-glucose levels because it affects hormones, which can increase blood-glucose levels. When we are "stressed out," the body releases many types of "flight or fight" hormones, which drive up blood-glucose and insulin levels. While it is unrealistic to expect to avoid stress, it's a good idea to minimize external causes of stress, and find some relaxation techniques to help reduce it. Yoga, meditation, craftwork, listening to music, and gardening are all good forms of relaxation techniques.

Alcohol Consumption While on the Diet

Straight spirits and dry red wines are optional while on a ketogenic diet. Please be aware that when one is in ketosis, alcohol can have a greater, faster effect. Moderation and self-experimentation are essential. Individuals will need to go slowly and monitor and assess the effects of alcohol on their blood-glucose and ketone levels, adjusting intake as effects are noted.

Be aware that alcohol has no nutrients and is a toxic substance that must be metabolized through the liver to detoxify and excrete it. When consumed in significant amounts (more than one drink per day), alcohol has adverse effects on the liver, and this is especially true for those with diabetes. This is in addition to the widely known adverse effects of alcohol on brain function and behavior. In addition, alcohol can result in worsening blood-sugar control, including hyperglycemia and hypoglycemia in persons with diabetes. Hypoglycemia can be precipitated by alcohol consumption without food. Heavy alcohol consumption without food can also cause alcoholic ketoacidosis.

Alcohol can by itself cause many of the same complications as diabetes and, of course, add to the risk of developing them in those with diabetes. Such complications include nerve damage, eye damage, heart disease, and high blood pressure.

A review paper titled "Consequences of Alcohol Use in Diabetics" provides additional details on the effects of alcohol ingestion in persons with diabetes. There are no significant health benefits from drinking alcohol, despite reports about the "antioxidant" polyphenols, like resveratrol, in red wine. Beers contain other nonalcoholic carbohydrates, as they are made from grain, and mixed drinks often contain sugar.

This is the bottom line: It is Dr. Runyan's opinion that the adverse effects of alcohol in persons with diabetes far exceed any potential health benefits and, therefore, alcohol consumption is not recommended.

Should one decide to drink alcohol, it should be no more than one drink on an occasional basis, and it should be taken with food, especially if you are following a ketogenic diet.

Ketone Supplementation

Ketone supplements are becoming more popular, and we are often asked about the use of these products. Although there is some research evidence that they are beneficial in the athletic performance world, as of 2017, no studies have been published which looked at the effects of these products for those with diabetes.

Some people have asked about using them during the transition period of adopting a ketogenic diet to minimize hypoglycemia. Theoretically, it is possible that ketone supplements could be used to guard against the symptoms of hypoglycemia, but this use has not been tested in controlled studies, so we have no data to say that it is valid. In addition, the effects of ketone supplementation only last a few hours, so they would need to be taken quite often to work. Since these products are expensive, the cost of this solution reduces its usefulness.

Ketone supplements elevate blood beta-hydroxybutyrate temporarily, but are a source of extra calories without any other nutrients. In persons without diabetes, exogenous ketones also lower blood glucose. Since they have not been tested in persons with diabetes, it is not possible to predict their effect on blood glucose. Hence, use of these products would need to be taken into account in relation to diabetic medications and insulin dosing, so that blood sugar is not inadvertently reduced to dangerous levels.

Skeptical Physicians and Diabetes Educators

If your physician or diabetes educator is skeptical about the efficacy of ketogenic diets for the treatment of diabetes, please give him or her a copy of a published review article titled "Dietary carbohydrate restriction as the first approach in diabetes management." This freely available paper was written by a team of the top low-carb experts and researchers, and it presents a twelve-point list of reasons why a low-carb diet is the logical treatment of choice for diabetes. It also refutes common misconceptions about the diet with strong science. The burden of proof is on the skeptic once this paper is read and understood.[10]

Resources for More Information

The following websites, videos and books are recommended as resources for obtaining more information about ketogenic diets and diabetes.

Website Resources

- Ellen's website: ketogenic-diet-resource.com
- Dr. Runyan's website: ketogenicdiabeticathlete.wordpress.com
- Dr. Richard Bernstein's website: www.diabetes-book.com
- Jeff Volek's YouTube talk on "The Many Facets of Keto-Adaptation": www.youtube.com/watch?v=GC1vMBRFiwE
- Kelley Pounds' Low Carb RN website: www.lowcarbrn.com
- Dr. Andreas Eenfeldt's website Diet Doctor: www.dietdoctor.com/diabetes
- Dr. Jay Wortman's My Big Fat Diet documentary on treating obesity, metabolic syndrome, and diabetes in a First Nation community: www.mybigfatdiet.net
- Jenny Ruhl's Diabetes 101 website: www.phlaunt.com
- David Mendosa's diabetes website: www.mendosa.com
- D-Solve diabetes website: dsolve.com
- Sandy Bahr's blog: ketodiabetes.blogspot.com

Recommended Books

- *Dr. Bernstein's Diabetes Solution* by Richard K. Bernstein, MD
- *The Diabetes Diet: Dr. Bernstein's Low-Carbohydrate Solution* by Richard K. Bernstein, MD
- *New Atkins for a New You: The Ultimate Diet for Shedding Weight and Feeling Great* by Eric Westman, MD; Jeff Volek, PhD, RD; and Stephen Phinney, MD, PhD
- *The Art and Science of Low Carbohydrate Living: An Expert's Guide to Making the Life-Saving Benefits of Carbohydrate Restriction Sustainable and Enjoyable* by Jeff Volek and Stephen Phinney

- *The Art and Science of Low Carbohydrate Performance* by Jeff Volek, PhD, RD; and Stephen Phinney, MD, PhD
- *Ketogenic Diets: Treatments for Epilepsy and Other Disorders* by John M. Freeman, MD; Eric Kossoff, MD; Zahava Turner, RD; and James E. Rubenstein, MD
- *Good Calories, Bad Calories* by Gary Taubes
- *Why We Get Fat: And What to Do About It* by Gary Taubes
- *Living Low Carb: Controlled-Carbohydrate Eating for Long-Term Weight Loss* by Jonny Bowden, PhD, CNS; and Barry Sears, PhD
- *The Low Carb Dietitian's Guide to Health and Beauty: How a Whole-Foods, Low-Carbohydrate Lifestyle Can Help You Look and Feel Better Than Ever* by Franziska Spritzler and Jacqueline A. Eberstein
- *Dr. Atkins' New Diet Revolution* by Robert C. Atkins, MD
- *Keto Clarity: Your Definitive Guide to the Benefits of a Low-Carb, High-Fat Diet* by Jimmy Moore and Eric Westman MD
- *The New Atkins Made Easy: A Faster, Simpler Way to Shed Weight and Feel Great—Starting Today!* by Colette Heimowitz
- *The Big Fat Surprise: Why Butter, Meat and Cheese Belong in a Healthy Diet* by Nina Teicholz
- *The Case Against Sugar* by Gary Taubes

Appendixes

Appendix A
Supplement Recommendations

Micronutrients are just as important as macronutrients. Micronutrients include vitamins, antioxidants, electrolytes, and minerals, and they are required in small quantities to support a range of physiological functions. These can be obtained from meat, organ meat, bone broth, fish, eggs, nuts, seeds, animal fats, tropical oils, non-starchy vegetables, and low-sugar fruits—all of which make up a ketogenic diet.

Although a balanced diet of real foods can provide many of the micronutrients needed, supplements can be helpful. Look for those with the lowest carbohydrate levels. Read labels to rule out those that contain sugar alcohols or other hidden carbohydrates. The following supplements are recommended:

- A carbohydrate-free multivitamin/mineral supplement. Make sure it contains at least 100% of the RDA for selenium and zinc. The Nature's Life Mighty Mini Vite Micro Tablet product offers just the minimal baseline coverage and is recommended.
- Vitamin D3 in the form of cholecalciferol, 2000 IU. The Country Life brand offers a gel-cap product with medium-chain triglycerides.
- Magnesium citrate, 400 mg daily, taken at bedtime if possible. You can also use a product called Natural Calm. It's a powder that can be mixed into a beverage and sipped throughout the day.
- CoQ10 (Ubiquinol or Ubiquinone), 100 mg daily.
- Now brand potassium chloride powder. It is very important to get enough potassium each day. Drinking homemade mineral water is one option, as is including green vegetables, small amounts of nuts, and plenty of avocadoes in your diet on a regular basis.
- CardiaSalt, Lite Salt, or NuSalt. You can find these salt substitutes at most grocery stores or on Amazon. You can use regular salt or these salt substitutes for flavoring your food.

- Homemade mineral water: Follow the recipe below EXACTLY, and sip this water only if you have symptoms such as fatigue, dizziness, or headaches. (See Possible Side Effect 3 in chapter 3.)

Homemade Mineral Water

To 1 quart of cold water add exactly 1/4 teaspoon of Now brand potassium chloride powder and exactly 1 level teaspoon of table or sea salt (provides sodium and chloride). Mix well and store in the refrigerator.

If you prefer not to take supplements, we have created a list of various nutrient-dense foods and the micronutrient amounts that each contains. You can download a document containing the Food Nutrient Lists from the "Resources" page on ketogenic-diet-resource.com.

Appendix B

Daily Protein Recommendations

These tables provide baseline minimum and maximum protein gram needs for most people based on the goal body weight.

Goal weight (lb.)	Goal weight (kg)	Minimum protein grams per day (1.0g/kg)	Maximum protein grams per day (1.5g/kg)
110	50	50	75
115	52	52	78
120	54	54	82
125	57	57	85
130	59	59	88
135	61	61	92
140	64	64	95
145	66	66	99
150	68	68	102
155	70	70	105
160	73	73	109
165	75	75	112
170	77	77	116
175	79	79	119
180	82	82	122
185	84	84	126
190	86	86	129
195	88	88	133
200	91	91	136
205	93	93	139
210	95	95	143
215	98	98	146
220	100	100	150
225	102	102	153
230	104	104	156
235	107	107	160
240	109	109	163
245	111	111	167
250	113	113	170
255	116	116	174
260	118	118	177
265	120	120	180
270	122	122	184
275	125	125	187
280	127	127	191
285	129	129	194
290	132	132	197

Appendix C
Food Lists

The food lists in this appendix are by no means comprehensive, but they should address most of the common foods suitable for a ketogenic diet. There are many online resources available, which contain thousands of food listings. We've recommended several in this book:

- Cronometer.com has a ketogenic option.
- Fitday.com offers both a web-based application and an application that can be downloaded to a PC.
- Myfitnesspal.com offers both a web-based and mobile application, and is another good choice, and it's free.
- The USDA's free nutrition database (http://ndb.nal.usda.gov).
- Atkins.com also has some tools for tracking progress on a ketogenic diet plan.

There are many food-count books on the market too:

- *The Calorie King* book gets good reviews on Amazon, and it comes in both a paperback and digital edition.
- *The Complete Book of Food Counts,* ninth edition, by Corrine Netzer.
- *Dana Carpender's Carb and Calorie Counter.*

The food lists begin on the next page.

Fat and Oil Foods

	Calories	Fat (g)	Carbs (g)	Fiber (g)	Protein (g)
Avocado oil, 1 tbsp.	124	14	0	0	0
Avocado, Haas, 3 oz.	102	9	7	5	2
Bacon fat, 1 tbsp.	116	13	0	0	0
Beef tallow, 1 tbsp.	115	13	0	0	0
Butter, 1 tbsp.	102	12	0	0	0
Chicken fat, 1 tbsp.	115	13	0	0	0
Cocoa butter, 1 tbsp.	120	14	0	0	0
Coconut oil, 1 tbsp.	117	14	0	0	0
Cream cheese (block), 2 tbsp.	101	10	1	0	2
Flaxseed oil, 1 tbsp.	120	14	0	0	0
Ghee, 1 tbsp.	112	13	0	0	0
Heavy cream, fluid, 2 tbsp.	103	11	1	0	1
Lard, fresh (non-hydrogenated), 1 tbsp.	115	13	0	0	0
Macadamia oil, 1 tbsp.	120	14	0	0	0
Mayonnaise (full-fat), 1 tbsp.	99	11	1	0	0
MCT oil, 1 tbsp.	100	14	0	0	0
Olive oil, 1 tbsp.	119	14	0	0	0
Red palm oil, 1 tbsp.	120	14	0	0	0
Salad dressing, creamy, full-fat (<2 carb/serving), 1.5 tbsp.	130	14	1	0	1
Sour cream (full-fat, no fillers, e.g., Daisy brand), 4 tbsp.	120	10	2	0	2

High-Fat, Moderate-Protein Combination Foods

	Calories	Fat (g)	Carbs (g)	Fiber (g)	Protein (g)
Almond meal (flour), 1 oz.	160	14	6	3	6
Cheese, feta, 3 oz.	120	11	3	1	6
Coconut butter, 2 tbsp.	186	18	8	4	2
Coconut, dried, unsweetened, 1 oz.	165	15	6	4	3
Nuts, almond, roasted, 1 oz.	172	16	5	3	6

Nuts, Brazil, roasted, 1 oz.	186	19	3	2	4
Nuts, cashew, 1 oz.	164	14	10	0	8
Nuts, hazelnut, 1 oz.	183	18	5	3	4
Nuts, macadamia, roasted, 1 oz.	203	22	4	3	2
Nuts, pecan, roasted, 1 oz.	201	21	4	3	3
Nuts, walnut, 1 oz.	185	18	4	2	4
Seeds, chia, 1 oz.	140	10	12	10	4
Seeds, flax, 1 oz.	152	12	8	7	6
Seeds, pumpkin, roasted, 1 oz.	148	12	4	1	9
Seeds, sesame, 1 oz.	161	14	7	5	5
Seeds, sunflower, roasted, 1 oz.	168	15	6	3	6

High-Protein, Moderate-Fat Foods

	Calories	Fat (g)	Carbs (g)	Fiber (g)	Protein (g)
Bacon, cooked, 2 slices	92	9	2	0	4
Beef, ground, 80% lean, cooked, 1 oz.	74	5	0	0	7
Cheese, blue, 1 oz.	100	8	1	0	6
Cheese, brie, 1 oz.	95	8	0	0	6
Cheese, cheddar, natural, 1 oz.	114	9	0	0	7
Cheese, Mexican blend, 1 oz.	105	9	1	0	7
Cheese, Monterey Jack, 1 oz.	106	9	0	0	7
Cheese, mozzarella, part skim, 1 oz.	72	5	1	0	7
Cheese, mozzarella, whole milk, 1 oz.	90	7	1	0	6
Cheese, parmesan, hard, 1 oz.	111	7	1	0	10
Cheese, provolone, 1 oz.	100	8	1	0	7
Cheese, ricotta, whole milk, 0.25 cup	107	8	2	0	7
Cheese, Swiss, 1 oz.	108	8	2	0	8
Duck, roasted, skin eaten, 1 oz.	95	8	0	0	5
Egg, whole, large, plain, 1 ea.	72	5	0	0	6
Lamb, boneless, cooked, 1 oz.	83	6	0	0	7
Pork sausage, cooked, 1.5 oz.	102	9	0	0	7

Pork ribs, roasted, plain, 1 oz.	104	8	0	0	8
Pork shoulder, roasted, 1 oz.	82	6	0	0	7
Yogurt, Greek, full-fat, 3.5 oz.	95	5	4	0	9

Lean-Protein Foods

	Calories	Fat (g)	Carbs (g)	Fiber (g)	Protein (g)
Beef, ground, 92% lean, cooked, 1 oz.	45	2	0	0	7
Beef steak, broiled or baked, 1 oz.	71	4	0	0	8
Beef, chuck, blade roast, cooked, 1 oz.	75	4	0	0	9
Chicken breast, roasted or baked, skin not eaten, 1 oz.	46	1	0	0	9
Chicken thigh, roasted, no skin, 1.0 oz.	55	3	0	0	7
Clams, fresh, baked, 1 oz.	39	2	1	0	4
Cottage cheese, 1% or 2%, 0.25 cup	41	1	2	0	7
Crab, king, fresh, steamed, 1.5 oz.	41	0	0	0	7.5
Egg whites, raw, large egg, 2 ea.	34	0	0	0	7
Elk steak, roasted, 1 oz.	41	.5	0	0	8.5
Fish fillet (flounder, sole, scrod), no breading, baked, 2 oz.	49	1	0	0	8.5
Fish, salmon fresh fillet, 1 oz.	39	1	0	0	7
Fish, salmon, canned, pink, 1 oz.	39	1	0	0	7
Ham, deli style, lean, 1 oz.	35	1	1	0	5
Ham, smoked, spiral, 1 oz.	53	3	1	0	5
Pork chops, lean, cooked, 1 oz.	57	3	0	0	7
Pork roast, loin, cooked, 1 oz.	70	4	0	0	8
Scallops, baked or broiled, 1 oz.	38	1	1	0	6
Shrimp, steamed or boiled, 1 oz.	39	1	0	0	8
Tuna, canned, water pack, 1 oz.	33	0	0	0	7
Turkey breast, roasted, no skin, 1 oz.	38	0	0	0	9
Turkey thigh, roasted, no skin, 1 oz.	52	2	0	0	8
Yogurt, Greek, 0% fat, 3 oz.	50	0	3.5	0	9

Carbohydrate Foods

	Calories	Fat (g)	Carbs (g)	Fiber (g)	Protein (g)
Asparagus, cooked, 1 cup	46	2	6	4	5
Beans, cooked (black, kidney) 0.25 cup	55	0	10	3	4
Beans, green, cooked, 1 cup	34	.5	8	4	2
Blueberries, raw, whole, 0.25 cup	21	0	5	1	0
Broccoli, cooked, chopped, 0.5 cup	27	0	6	3	2
Brussels sprouts, raw, 1 cup	38	0	8	3	3
Cabbage, green, raw, shredded, 4 oz.	23	0	5	2	1
Carrots, baby, raw, 2 oz.	20	0	6	2	0
Cauliflower, cooked, 1 cup	28	0	6	2	2
Celery, raw, chopped, 1 cup	36	0	7	4	2
Chickpeas, cooked, ¼ cup	67	1	11	3	4
Cucumber, raw, sliced, 10 oz.	29	0	6	2	1
Eggplant, raw, 6 oz.	33	0	8	5	1
Garlic, 6 cloves	24	0	6	0	0
Green beans, cooked, 0.5 cup	22	0	5	1	1
Kale, raw, chopped, 2 oz.	28	0	6	1	2
Lemon juice, 1 tbsp.	3	0	1	0	0
Lettuce, any leaf, shredded, 3 cups	24	0	6	3	3
Lettuce, iceberg, shredded, 3 cups	24	0	6	3	0
Lettuce, romaine shredded, 3 cups	24	0	6	3	3
Lime juice, 1 tbsp.	3	0	1	0	0
Mushrooms, button, raw, 6 oz.	37	1	6	2	5
Mushrooms, portabella, raw, 4 oz.	29	0	6	2	3
Onion, green, 0.5 cup	16	0	4	1	1
Onion, white, raw, 0.5 cup	33	0	7	1	1
Pepper, bell, raw, 4 oz.	23	0	5	2	0
Potato, white, cooked, 0.5 cup	95	4	13	2	1
Raspberries, raw, whole, 0.5 cup	32	0	7	4	1
Rice, white, cooked, 0.25 cup	51	0	11	0	1
Shallots, chopped, 2 tbsp.	14	0	4	0	0

Spinach, cooked, from frozen, 5 oz.	57	3	5	3	4
Spinach, raw, 6 oz.	38	1	6	4	1
Squash, spaghetti, cooked, 1 cup	75	0	10	2	1
Squash, summer, cooked, sliced, 1 cup	36	0	8	3	2
Strawberries, raw, whole, 0.5 cup	23	0	6	2	0
Swiss chard, chopped coarse, 3 cups	21	0	4	2	2
Tomato sauce, 0.5 cup	40	0	8	2	2
Tomato, raw, 6 oz.	31	0	7	2	1
Turnips, raw, 4 oz.	32	0	7	2	1

Miscellaneous Foods (add your own)

	Calories	Fat (g)	Carbs (g)	Fiber (g)	Protein (g)
Olives, black, 1 cup	141	13	8	4	1
Olives, green, 1 cup	193	20	5	4	1
Pork rinds, fried, 0.75 oz.*	116	7	0	0	13*

*Note on pork rinds: The protein in this food is inferior in quality. Count the protein grams but limit amounts eaten so as not to displace other more complete protein foods.

Spice Carb Counts

Spice	Carbs in 1 tbsp.
Allspice, ground	3.0
Basil, dried	0.9
Black pepper	2.4
Caraway seed	0.8
Cardamom, ground	2.4
Cayenne pepper	1.6
Cinnamon, ground	1.7
Cloves	1.7
Coriander seed	0.6
Cumin, ground	2.1
Curry powder	1.6
Fennel seed	0.7
Garlic powder	5.3
Ginger, ground	3.1
Imitation vanilla extract	0.3
Mace, ground	1.6
Nutmeg	2.0
Onion powder	5.2
Oregano, ground	0.4
Paprika	1.2
Parsley, dried	0.3
Peppermint, fresh	0.1
Poppy seeds	1.2
Poultry seasoning	2.0
Pumpkin-pie spice	3.1
Sage, ground	0.4
Spearmint, dried	0.3
Tarragon, ground	2.0
Thyme, ground	1.1
Vanilla extract	1.6
White pepper	3.0

Appendix D
Conversions and Measurements

Rules for Measures
- Multiply grams by 0.0353 to get the weight in ounces.
- Multiply ounces by 28.35 to get the weight in grams.

Dry Measure Equivalents

Measurement →	Equal to →	Equal to →	Equal to
3 teaspoons	1 tablespoon	1/2 ounce	14.3 grams
2 tablespoons	1/8 cup	1 ounce	28.3 grams
4 tablespoons	1/4 cup	2 ounces	56.7 grams
5 1/3 tablespoons	1/3 cup	2.6 ounces	75.6 grams
8 tablespoons	1/2 cup	4 ounces	113.4 grams
12 tablespoons	3/4 cup	6 ounces	169.8 grams
32 tablespoons	2 cups	16 ounces	452.8 grams

Volume (Liquid) Measurements

American cups and quarts equal to →	American ounces equal to →	Metric (milliliters and liters)
2 tbsp.	1 fl. oz.	30 ml
¼ cup	2 fl. oz.	60 ml
½ cup	4 fl. oz.	125 ml
1 cup	8 fl. oz.	250 ml
1 ½ cups	12 fl. oz.	375 ml
2 cups or 1 pint	16 fl. oz.	500 ml
4 cups or 1 quart	32 fl. oz.	1000 ml or 1 liter
1 gallon	128 fl. oz.	4 liters

Oven Temperatures

Fahrenheit	Celsius
250° F	130° C
300° F	150° C
350° F	180° C
400° F	200° C
450° F	230° C

Abbreviations

Abbrev.	Full term
ea.	each
oz.	ounce
tbsp.	tablespoon
tsp.	teaspoon

Ketone Conversion Formula

The exact calculation rule is shown here:

[Value in mg/dL] is divided by 10.41	mmol/L
[Value in mmol/L] multiplied by 10.41	mg/dL

The easier method:

[Value in mg/dL] divided by 10	mmol/L
[Value in mmol/L] multiplied by 10	mg/dL

Blood-Glucose Conversion Formula

The exact calculation rule shown below:

[Value in mg/dL] multiplied by 0.0555	mmol/L
[Value in mmol/L] multiplied by 18.0182	mg/dL

The easier method:

[Value in mg/dL] divided by 18	mmol/L
[Value in mmol/L] multiplied by 18	mg/dL

Blood-Glucose Conversion Table: mg/dL to mmol

mg/dL	mmol
50	3.0
55	3.1
60	3.3
65	3.6
70	3.9
75	4.2
80	4.4
85	4.7
90	5.0
95	5.3
100	5.6
105	5.8
110	6.1
115	6.4
120	6.7
125	6.9
130	7.2
135	7.5
140	7.8
145	8.1
150	8.3
155	8.6
160	8.9
165	9.2
170	9.4
175	9.7
180	10.0
185	10.3

Hemoglobin A1c (HbA1c) to Average Blood-Glucose Conversion

HbA1C	Average Blood Glucose	
	mg/dL	mmol/l
4.5	82	4.6
5	96	5.4
5.5	111	6.2
6	125	6.9
6.5	140	7.7
7	155	8.5
7.5	169	9.3
8	184	10.1
8.5	197	10.9
9	214	11.7
9.5	226	12.6
10	240	13.3
10.5	254	14.1
11	269	14.9
11.5	283	15.7
12	298	16.5
12.5	312	17.3
13	326	18.1
14	355	19.7
15	383	21.3
16	413	22.9
17	441	24.5

Appendix E
Legal Disclaimer and Terms of Use

This Legal Disclaimer and Terms of Use Agreement is entered into between Ellen Davis and Keith Runyan, MD, the authors of this document, the Ketogenic Diet Resource website and you. All of the information provided in and throughout this book (hereafter known as Publication) or offered at http://www.Ketogenic-Diet-Resource.com are intended solely for general information and should NOT be relied upon for any particular diagnosis, treatment, or care. This is not a substitute for medical advice or treatment. This Publication is only for general informational purposes. It is strongly encouraged that individuals and their families consult with qualified medical professionals for treatment and related advice on individual cases before beginning any diet. Decisions relating to the prevention, detection, and treatment of all health issues should be made only after discussing the risks and benefits with your health care provider, taking into account your personal medical history, your current situation, and your future health risks and concerns. If you are pregnant, nursing, diabetic, on medication, have a medical condition, or are beginning a health or weight-control program, consult your physician before using products or services discussed in this book and before making any other dietary changes. The authors and publisher cannot guarantee that the information in this Publication is safe and proper for every reader. For this reason, this Publication is sold without warranties or guarantees of any kind, express or implied, and the authors and publisher disclaim any liability, loss, or damage caused by the contents, either directly or consequentially. Neither the US Food and Drug Administration nor any other government regulatory body has evaluated statements made in this Publication. Products, services, and methods discussed in this Publication are not intended to diagnose, treat, cure, or prevent any disease.

Indemnification:

All users of this book agree to defend, indemnify, and hold harmless Ketogenic-Diet-Resource.com, its contributors, any entity jointly created by them, their respective affiliates and their respective directors, officers, employees, and agents from and against all claims and expenses, including attorneys' fees, arising out of the use of this Publication.

Disclaimer of Liability:

Neither Ketogenic-Diet-Resource.com nor its contributors shall be held liable for any use of the information described and/or contained herein and assumes no responsibility for anyone's use of the information. In no event shall the Ketogenic-Diet-Resource.com website or its contributors be liable for any direct, indirect, incidental, special, exemplary, or consequential damages (including but not limited to: procurement of substitute goods or services; loss of use, data, or profits; or business interruption) however caused and on any theory of liability, whether in contract, strict liability, tort (including negligence or otherwise), or any other theory arising in any way out of the use of this material, even if Ketogenic-Diet-Resource.com has been advised of the possibility of such damage. This disclaimer of liability applies to any damages or injury, whether based on alleged breach of contract, tortious behavior, negligence, or any other cause of action, including but not limited to damages or injuries caused by any failure of performance, error, omission, interruption, deletion, defect, delay in operation or transmission, computer virus, communication line failure, and/or theft, destruction, or unauthorized access to, alteration of, or use of any record.

Rules of Conduct: No Warranties:

All content in this Publication is provided to you on an "as is," "as available" basis without warranty of any kind, either express or implied, including but not limited to the implied warranties of merchantability, fitness for a particular purpose, and non-infringement. Ketogenic-Diet-Resource.com makes no warranty as to the accuracy, completeness, currency, or reliability of any content available through this website. Ketogenic-Diet-Resource.com makes no representations, or warranties of any kind, that use of the website will be uninterrupted or error-free. The user is responsible for taking all precautions necessary to ensure that any web-based content offered from the website or Publication is free of viruses.

Limitation of Liability:

Ketogenic-Diet-Resource.com specifically disclaims any and all liability, whether based in contract, tort, strict liability or otherwise, for any direct, indirect, incidental, consequential, or special damages arising out of or in any way connected with access to or use of the website or Publication even if Ketogenic-Diet-Resource.com has been advised of the possibility of such damages. This limitation of liability includes, but is not limited to, reliance by any party on any content obtained through use of this website, or that arises in connection with mistakes or omissions in, or delays in transmission of information to or from the user, interruptions in telecommunications connections to this website, this Publication, or viruses, whether caused in whole or in part by negligence, acts of God, telecommunications failure, theft or destruction of or unauthorized access to the website, Publication, or related information.

Modifications:

Ketogenic-Diet-Resource.com reserves the right to modify this Publication and the rules and regulations governing its use at any time. Modifications will be posted on the website, and users are deemed to be apprised of and bound by any changes to the website. Your continued use of this Publication following the posting of changes to these Terms of Use constitutes your acceptance of those changes. Ketogenic-Diet-Resource.com may make changes in the products and/or services described in this Publication at any time.

Governing Law, Forum Selection, and General Provisions:

This Publication was created and uploaded by Ketogenic-Diet-Resource.com from its place of business in Wyoming, USA. Ketogenic-Diet-Resource.com makes no representation that the information in the Publication is appropriate or available for use in other locations. Access to the Publication from territories where the contents of the Publication may be illegal is prohibited. Those who choose to access this Publication from other locations do so at their own initiative and are responsible for compliance with applicable local laws. This Agreement shall be governed by and interpreted in accordance with the laws of Wyoming, USA, excluding the application of its conflicts of law rules, and all claims relating or arising out of this Agreement, whether sounding in contract, tort or otherwise, shall likewise be governed by the laws of Wyoming, USA, excluding the application of its conflicts of law rules. You agree that all actions or proceedings arising in connection with this Agreement shall be tried and litigated exclusively in the state and federal courts located in the County of Laramie, State of Wyoming, USA. The aforementioned choice of venue is intended to be mandatory and not permissive in nature, thereby precluding the possibility of litigation with respect to or arising out of this Agreement in any jurisdiction other than that specified in this paragraph. You agree that the state and federal courts located in the County of Laramie, State of Wyoming shall have in personam jurisdiction and venue over you for the purpose of litigating any dispute, controversy, or proceeding arising out of or related to this Agreement.

Severability

If a section of this disclaimer is determined by any court or other competent authority to be unlawful and/or unenforceable, the other sections of this disclaimer shall continue in effect.

References

Glossary

Acetoacetate (AcAc)   A water soluble ketone body produced by the liver from the metabolism of fatty acids when carbohydrate intake is restricted and glycogen stores are low or the body is in a fasted state. It can be used as a fuel source by most normal cells in the body when blood-glucose availability is low. Acetoacetate can be converted into two other ketone bodies, beta-hydroxybutyrate and acetone. See also *ketone body, acetone* and *beta-hydroxybutyrate*.

Acetone   One of the three types of ketone bodies, acetone is a spontaneous byproduct of the breakdown of acetoacetate. Acetone is expelled from the body via the breath.

Acidosis   Acidosis is a condition in which the blood is too acidic (blood pH falls below 7.35), which manifests in the symptoms of rapid breathing, confusion or lethargy. It can be fatal if not treated.

ADA   American Diabetes Association

Adipose   Fat tissue in the body.

Adiposity   Measure of the amount of body fat.

Adrenalin   See *epinephrine*. Also called the "fight or flight" response hormone. It is released from neurons and the adrenal glands in response to various stimuli (exercise, low blood glucose, fear) and results in a release of glucose into the bloodstream, increased blood flow to the muscles, increased heart rate and other metabolic effects.

Advanced glycation end-products (AGEs)   Body proteins or fats that become glycated after exposure to sugars. AGEs are the common cause of diabetic complications. The presence and accumulation of AGEs in many different cell types affect extracellular and intracellular structure and function. Also see *glycation*.

Aerobic exercise   Sustained, cadenced exercise that increases your heart rate; also referred to as cardio.

AGEs   See *advanced glycation end-products* and *glycation*.

Agonist   A substance that acts like another substance and therefore stimulates an action.

Alpha cell   Specialized cell in the pancreatic Islet of Langerhans that produces glucagon when the body needs it.

Amino acids   The molecular building blocks of proteins. There are over 300 different amino acids in nature. Humans depend on twenty different amino acids and eight of those are essential, meaning they have to be obtained from the diet.

Amylin   A hormone cosecreted with insulin by the beta cells of the pancreas that inhibits glucagon, delays emptying of the stomach, and acts to increase satiety.

Anoxic   Total depletion in the level of oxygen.

Antioxidants   Substances that neutralize harmful free radicals and reactive oxygen species.

Apoptosis   The metabolic process of programmed cell death. In normal cells, apoptosis is triggered when a cell is damaged to minimize toxic releases to surrounding cells. Cancer cells tend to have defective mechanisms to trigger apoptosis.

Arrhythmia   Any of a group of conditions in which the heartbeat is irregular or is faster or slower than normal.

Asymptomatic   Having no symptoms.

Atherosclerosis   Clogging, narrowing, and hardening of blood vessels by plaque deposits.

ATP   Adenosine triphosphate. A molecule that transports chemical energy within cells for metabolic purposes.

Basal insulin   The role of basal insulin, also known as background insulin, is to keep blood glucose at consistent levels during periods of fasting. Basal insulin has to act over a relatively long period of time and, therefore, will be either long-acting insulin or intermediate insulin.

Baseline blood sugar   The blood-sugar measurement before insulin or a meal is given.

Beta cells (β-cells)   Specialized cells in the pancreas that produce the hormones insulin and amylin.

Beta-hydroxybutyrate (BOHB)   A ketone body generated from the conversion of acetoacetate, the main ketone body produced by the liver from the metabolism of fatty acids when carbohydrate intake is restricted and glycogen stores are low or the body is in a fasted state. See also *acetone* and *acetoacetate*.

Blood glucose (sugar)   The amount of glucose or sugar in the bloodstream at any one time.

Blood lipids   The medical term for the total cholesterol, triglycerides, and HDL and LDL cholesterol in your blood.

Blood pressure   The pressure your blood exerts against the walls of your arteries during a heartbeat.

Body mass index (BMI)   A measure of body fat based on height and weight for adults.

Bolus insulin   A bolus dose of insulin is specifically taken at mealtimes to keep blood-glucose levels under control following a meal. Bolus insulin needs to act quickly and so short-acting insulin or rapid-acting insulin will be used.

Branched chain amino acids (BCAA)   BCAAs are a category of three specific amino acids: isoleucine, leucine and valine. They function in the body to ramp up protein synthesis and provide energy. Leucine especially has been shown to stimulate tumor growth.

Carb-adaptation   The process of becoming adapted to using carbohydrates and glucose as the main cellular fuel.

Carbohydrate (carb)   Foods that are broken down by digestion into simple sugars, such as glucose, to provide a source of energy. Examples are starches, such as potatoes, wheat, rice and corn, and sweet foods, such as sugar, candy, juice, cakes, pies, cookies and ice cream.

Cellular respiration   The process that all cells use to produce energy. It involves both glucose and oxygen and involves cellular mitochondria.

Cerebrovascular   Pertaining to the blood vessels and, especially, the arteries that supply the brain.

CGM   Continuous glucose monitor. Also known as real-time continuous glucose monitor (rt-CGM). A device with a tiny glucose sensor that is inserted under the skin to measure glucose levels in tissue fluid after it has been calibrated initially and every twelve hours thereafter using a blood-glucose meter reading.

Cholesterol   A waxy substance essential for many of the body's functions, including manufacturing hormones and making cell membranes.

Cortisol   A steroid hormone that is produced by the adrenal glands. It is released in response to stress and a low level of blood glucose. Its functions are to increase blood sugar through gluconeogenesis, to suppress the immune system, and to aid the metabolism of fat, protein and carbohydrate.

CRP   C-reactive protein is a protein produced by the liver in response to inflammation. See also *high-sensitivity C-reactive protein.*

CSII   A device that delivers a continuous subcutaneous insulin infusion, also known as an insulin pump.

CVD   Cardiovascular disease, also known as "hardening of the arteries" or heart disease.

Dawn phenomenon   A rise in blood-sugar levels in the early morning hours.

Diabetes   See *TD1M* and *T2DM (type 2 diabetes).*

Diabetic gastroparesis   Gastroparesis is a disorder affecting people with both type 1 and type 2 diabetes in which the stomach takes too long to empty its contents. It can make diabetes worse by making it more difficult to manage blood glucose.

Diabetic ketoacidosis (DKA)   A life-threatening condition associated with insulin deficiency and causing high blood sugar, dehydration, and an excess of ketone bodies, which render blood pH acidic. Treatment consists of emergency fluid and insulin treatment.

Diet-heart hypothesis   The hypothesis that a high intake of saturated fat and elevated LDL cholesterol are the most important causes of atherosclerosis and coronary heart disease. Also known as the lipid-heart hypothesis.

Diuretic   Any substance that causes fluid to be eliminated from the body by increasing urination.

Dyslipidemia   An elevation of plasma cholesterol, triglycerides (TGs), or both, or a low high-density lipoprotein level that contributes to the development of atherosclerosis. Diagnosis is made by measuring plasma levels of total cholesterol, TGs, and individual lipoproteins.

Endogenous   Sourced from within the body; having an internal cause or origin.

Epidemiological   Sourced in epidemiology, the science that studies the patterns, causes, and effects of health and disease conditions in defined populations. It is the

cornerstone of public health and informs policy decisions and evidence-based practice by identifying risk factors for disease and targets for preventive healthcare.

Epinephrine   More commonly known as adrenaline; a hormone secreted by the sympathetic nervous system and adrenal glands in response to low blood sugar when
insufficient ketones are available. It causes an increase in blood glucose by release
of glucose from the liver and kidneys and also causes symptoms of increased heart
rate and blood pressure.

Essential fatty acids (EFAs)   Two classes of essential dietary fats that must be obtained
from food or supplements. The two classes are Omega 3 and Omega 6, with the
numbers designating the location of the first chemical double bond in the molecule.

Essential nutrients   Essential nutrients are nutrients that are required for life that the
body cannot make internally. Hence, they must be obtained from the diet.

Exogenous   Sourced from outside the body; relating to, or developing from external
factors.

Fat   One of the three macronutrients; an organic compound that dissolves in other oils
but not in water. A source of energy and building blocks of cells. Foods rich in
fatty acids. There are three main types of fats found in food. Saturated fats are solid
at room temperature and include butter, coconut oil, ghee, lard and beef tallow.
Monounsaturated fats include olive oil. Polyunsaturated fats include vegetable oils
such as safflower, sunflower and soybean oil.

Fat-adaptation   See *keto-adaptation.*

Fatty acids   The scientific term for fat molecules in the body, which are part of a group of
substances called lipids. Fatty acids come in different lengths from 6 carbon to 26
carbon chains.

Fiber   Parts of plant foods that are indigestible or very slowly digested, with little effect
on blood sugar and insulin levels; sometimes called roughage. There are two types:
soluble and insoluble.

Free radicals   Chemically unstable molecules that "steal" electrons from surrounding
molecules. They are in the environment and naturally produced by our bodies.
Excess free radicals can damage cells through oxidative activity. Think of what rust
is to steel.

Fructosamine   Fructosamine is a molecule formed from the joining of fructose to protein
molecules in the blood through glycation. Tests for fructosamine are done when
hemoglobin anomalies render the hemoglobin A1c test inconclusive.

Fructose   A simple sugar found naturally in fruits and plants. It is also found in commercial sweeteners such as high-fructose corn syrup and crystalline fructose. Excess
intake of fructose has been implicated in many health issues.

GERD   Gastrointestinal-esophageal reflux disease. A medical term for severe heartburn.

Glucagon   A hormone secreted by the alpha cells of the pancreas that signals the liver
to break down stored glycogen into glucose and release it into the bloodstream to
maintain normal blood-sugar levels. Glucagon signaling is impaired in persons

with T1DM or advanced T2DM because beta-cell insulin secretion is the prime regulator of glucagon secretion. This impaired glucagon signaling translates to inadequate glucagon secretion during hypoglycemia and inadequate raising of blood glucose and unsuppressed glucagon secretion after meals, and this contributes to postprandial hyperglycemia.

Gluconeogenesis   The process by which glucose is formed in the liver from a non-carbohydrate source when blood sugar is low.

Glucose   A simple sugar that your cells use to make energy. It is created from the breakdown or metabolism of foods that contain carbohydrate (starches and sugars) and, to a lesser extent, protein foods such as meat and eggs.

Glucose intolerance   Abnormal increase in blood glucose after a carbohydrate containing meal or during an oral glucose-tolerance test (OGTT).

Glycation   A process in which excess blood glucose bonds or "sticks" to protein or fat molecules in body tissues, causing impairment of the glycated tissue. For example, nerve endings can become glycated and result in diabetic neuropathy (nerve pain). Glycation is like rubbing maple syrup on your hands and then trying to fold clothes or type on a keyboard.

Glycemic index   A measure of the blood-sugar increase after consuming a food containing 50 grams of carbohydrate compared to the blood-sugar increase from consuming 50 grams of glucose or white bread. The higher the glycemic index of a particular food, the higher the blood-sugar rise in response to consuming that food.

Glycemic load   The mathematical product of glycemic index and total carbohydrate content of a given food.

Glycerol   Glycerol is the "backbone" of a fatty acid or triglyceride. Imagine a capital *E*. The glycerol molecule represents the vertical spine of the *E* with fatty acids making up the horizontal lines of the *E*.

Glycogen   The storage form of carbohydrate in the body.

Glycolysis   The pathway by which glucose is broken down in the cell into two molecules of pyruvic acid with the generation of energy in the form of ATP.

Goal body weight (GBW)   The weight you would like to attain, or the weight at which you feel best.

HbA1c   Also known as glycated hemoglobin A1c, this is a test that measures average blood sugar over the past three months. It indicates to what level and time blood sugars have been elevated, because it measures the amount of "glycated" hemoglobin in red blood cells.

HDL cholesterol   High-density lipoprotein; the "good" type of cholesterol.

Hepatic   Coming from or having to do with the liver.

HFCS   High-fructose corn syrup. Cheap sweetener used in soft drinks and other processed food products.

HHS   Hyperglycemic hyperosmolar syndrome. HHS is the initial manifestation of diabetes in 7%–17% of patients. Infection is the major precipitating factor, occurring in 30%–60% of patients.

HIIT　High-intensity interval training. A type of exercise that is beneficial for improving insulin sensitivity.

Homocysteine　An amino acid that acts as a marker for heart disease. A high level of homocysteine in the blood (hyperhomocysteinemia) makes a person more prone to endothelial cell injury and inflammation in the blood vessels. This can increase the risk of atherosclerosis and heart attack.

High-sensitivity C-Reactive protein (hs-CRP)　A test that measures inflammation in the body. Inflammation is a marker for tissue damage that can be caused by elevated blood glucose.

Hydrogenated oils　Vegetable oils processed to solid form to improve their shelf life. See *trans fats*.

Hyperglycemia　A metabolic state of elevated blood sugar, which can cause body damage through the actions of glycation.

Hyperinsulinemia　Condition of chronically elevated blood-insulin levels.

Hypertension　Medical term for high blood pressure. Blood pressure is a measurement of the force of blood against your blood vessels, and it is reported as two numbers (e.g., 140/90). The top number is the systolic pressure, which is a measure of pressure in the arteries when the heart beats and pushes more blood into the arteries. The second number, called the diastolic pressure, is the pressure in the arteries when the heart rests between beats. The ideal blood pressure for non-pregnant people with diabetes is 130/80 or less.

Hypoglycemia　A metabolic state of low blood sugar. Hypoglycemia can be associated with symptoms such as rapid heart rate, profuse sweating, flushing, and confusion. It can also occur without symptoms, meaning that even though the measurement of blood sugar is low, no symptoms of low blood sugar are evident. The symptoms are caused by the brain's signal to the sympathetic nervous system and adrenal glands to release adrenaline (epinephrine), norepinephrine (the "fight or flight" hormone), and acetylcholine. These hormones normally signal the liver to break down stored sugar and release it into the bloodstream and to signal the person to seek out food, in particular, glucose. When the symptoms of hypoglycemia are either impaired or absent, it can be dangerous since the warning system is also absent. See hypoglycemia-associated autonomic failure (HAAF).

Hypoglycemia-associated autonomic failure (HAAF)　HAAF occurs most commonly in persons with T1DM or advanced insulin-deficient T2DM who have experienced recent hypoglycemic episodes during sleep or after exercise. These episodes cause both defective glucose-counter regulation (in the absence of decrements in insulin and increments in glucagon) and hypoglycemic unawareness (reduction in the sympathoadrenal responses) and, therefore, a vicious cycle of recurrent hypoglycemia.

Hypoglycemic unawareness　A reduction in the sympathoadrenal response to low blood sugar. It is a complication of diabetes in which the patient is unaware of a deep drop in blood sugar because it fails to trigger the secretion of epinephrine which generates the characteristic symptoms of hypoglycemia (such as palpitations, sweating, anxiety) that serve to warn the patient of the dropping blood-sugar levels.

Hyperglycemic hyperosmolar syndrome (HHS) Diabetic hyperglycemic hyperosmolar syndrome (HHS) is a complication of type 2 diabetes. It is characterized by extremely high blood-sugar levels without the presence of ketones.

Inflammation Part of the body's delicately balanced natural defense system against potentially damaging substances. Excessive inflammation is associated with increased risk of heart attack, stroke, diabetes, and some forms of cancer.

Islet cell Specialized cells in the pancreas that produce various endocrine hormones such as insulin, glucagon, somatostatin, ghrelin, and amylin.

Insulin Insulin is a hormone produced by the pancreas that signals cells to take up glucose and amino acids from the bloodstream. Insulin also blocks the release of fat from fat cells. Insulin is sourced and released from the pancreas (endogenous insulin) in proportion to the amount of glucose in the bloodstream. Insulin can also come from external or exogenous sources, such as insulin injections or pumps.

Insulin-like growth factor 1 (IGF-1) A hormone secreted by the liver; it is similar in structure to insulin. IGF-1 is one of the most potent natural activators of the AKT signaling pathway, a stimulator of cell growth and proliferation and a potent inhibitor of programmed cell death.

Insulinogenic Relating to or causing the stimulation of the production of insulin.

Insulin resistance (IR) A metabolic condition in which chronically high levels of circulating insulin result in body cells becoming desensitized and unable to respond properly to the insulin signal. Insulin's job is to push glucose from the bloodstream into cells where it can be metabolized for energy. Without proper insulin signaling, glucose builds up in the blood, which then perpetuates further elevation of insulin levels. If left untreated, this circle of insulin and glucose elevation can lead to a diagnosis of metabolic syndrome, prediabetes and can develop into type 2 diabetes (T2DM).

Keto-adaptation The process of becoming adapted to using ketones instead of glucose as the primary cellular fuel in the body. Also known as fat-adaptation.

Ketoacidosis The uncontrolled overproduction of ketones characteristic of untreated type 1 diabetes, with ketones typically five to ten times higher than in nutritional ketosis.

Ketogenesis The metabolic process in which the liver creates ketone bodies from the breakdown of fatty acids. The ketone bodies can then be metabolized within the cell mitochondria to fuel the body.

Ketogenic diet (KD) A high-fat, moderate-protein, low-carbohydrate diet used to treat various illnesses and improve health through a change in cellular fuel metabolism.

Ketone body A water soluble molecule produced by the liver from fatty acids during periods of low food intake (fasting) or carbohydrate restriction. They are used as an alternate energy source by various body cells and systems when glucose levels are low. The three ketone bodies are acetoacetate, beta-hydroxybutyrate and acetone.

Ketosis   A metabolic state where most of the body's energy supply comes from ketone bodies in the blood.

Lactose   The simple sugar (carbohydrate) found in milk and milk products such as cheese and yogurt. It has a pronounced effect on insulin.

LADA   The short term for latent autoimmune diabetes of adults. It is also called type 1.5 diabetes. A form of diabetes similar to type 1 diabetes, but it has a slow time period of development and so manifests in adulthood.

LCHF   Low-carb, high fat.

LDL cholesterol   Low-density lipoprotein. Commonly known as the "bad" type of cholesterol. However, only the small, dense LDL particles, which are associated with CVD, are "bad." Small, dense LDL particles occur in persons with insulin resistance consuming refined carbohydrates.

Lean body mass (LBM)   Body mass minus fat tissue; includes muscle, bone, organs, and connective tissue.

Legumes   Most members of the bean and pea families, including lentils, chickpeas, soybeans, and peas.

Lipid-heart hypothesis   The hypothesis that high intake of saturated fat and elevated LDL cholesterol are the most important causes of atherosclerosis and coronary heart disease. Also known as the diet-heart hypothesis.

Lipids   Lipids constitute a group of naturally occurring molecules that include fats, waxes, sterols such as cholesterol, fat-soluble vitamins (vitamins A, D, E and K), monoglycerides, diglycerides, triglycerides, phospholipids, and others. The main biological functions of lipids include energy storage, signaling, and acting as structural components of cell membranes.

Lipoprotein (a)   Lipoprotein (a), also known as Lp(a), is a subclass of LDL cholesterol. High Lp(a) blood levels are a risk factor for coronary heart disease (CHD), stroke, atherosclerosis, and thrombosis. High Lp(a) levels also predict risk of early atherosclerosis independently of other cardiac risk factors, including LDL.

Lumen   The inside space of a tubular structure within the body. For instance, the spinal cord is in the lumen of the spinal bone column.

Macronutrients   The three main types of nutrients in the diet: fat, protein and carbohydrate.

Macrophages   A type of white blood cell that engulfs and digests cellular debris, foreign substances, microbes, and cancer cells in an immune system process called phagocytosis.

Medium-chain triglycerides (MCTs)   MCTs are fatty acids with 6 to 10 carbon atoms that are more rapidly absorbed from the intestine compared to long-chain triglycerides. In addition, MCTs do not require intestinal bile salts for digestion. Individuals who have malnutrition or digestive absorption issues are treated with

MCTs because they don't require energy for absorption and utilization in the body, and they increase ketone production, especially in those following a ketogenic diet.

Multi-dose injections (MDI) Multiple-dose injection (MDI) therapy, also known as multiple daily injections, is an alternate term for the basal/bolus regime of injecting insulin. The therapy involves injecting a long-acting insulin once or twice daily as a background (basal) dose and having further injections of rapid-acting insulin at each mealtime.

Metabolic syndrome A group of conditions, including hypertension, high triglycerides, low HDL cholesterol, higher-than-normal blood-sugar and insulin levels, and weight carried in the middle of the body. Also known as syndrome X or insulin-resistance syndrome, it predisposes you to various diseases.

Metabolism The complex chemical processes that convert food into energy or the body's building blocks, which, in turn, become part of organs, tissues and cells.

mg/dL Stands for milligrams per deciliter. It's a unit of measure that shows the concentration of a substance in a specific amount of fluid. It is used as a standard measurement of blood sugar in test results.

Mitochondria Cell organelles, called the "cellular power plants" because they generate most of the cell's supply of adenosine triphosphate (ATP), the main form of cellular energy.

mM or mmol/L Stands for millimolar. A unit of measurement that represents a concentration of one thousandth of a solute mole per liter. Ketone levels in blood can be measured and reported in mM.

Monounsaturated fatty acids (MUFA) A type of dietary fat typically found in foods such as olive oil, canola oil, nuts, and avocados, and also beef steak.

Monosodium glutamate (MSG) Monosodium glutamate is a chemical used to heighten taste sensations in processed foods. MSG is a neurotoxin and should be avoided on a ketogenic diet because it contains glutamate, a derivate of glutamine.

Myocardial infarction Medical term for a heart attack that occurs when blood flow to the heart is compromised and the lack of oxygen injures the heart muscle.

Myocardium The muscular tissue of the heart.

NAFLD See nonalcoholic fatty liver disease.

Nephropathy Kidney disease; damage or disease that affects the kidneys.

Neuropathy Damage to or disease affecting nerves, which may impair sensation, movement, gland or organ function, or other aspects of health, depending on the type of nerve affected. See also *peripheral neuropathy.*

Nonalcoholic fatty liver disease (NAFLD) Nonalcoholic fatty liver disease (NAFLD) is the buildup of extra fat in the liver. NAFLD is associated with insulin resistance and metabolic syndrome and tends to develop more readily when the diet is high in sugars and fructose and low in choline.

Nutrient A nutrient is a chemical that an organism needs to live and grow. They are used to build and repair tissues and regulate body processes and are converted to and used as energy. For humans, fats, proteins, carbohydrates, vitamins, minerals, and water are the main nutrients.

Nutritional ketosis   The moderate and controlled level of ketones in the bloodstream that allows the body to function well with little dietary carbohydrate. A state of ketosis that is safe and normal when carbohydrate or calories are restricted.

OGTT   Oral glucose-tolerance test. A medical test in which a large amount of glucose is given and blood samples are taken afterward to determine how quickly the glucose is cleared from the blood.

Omega-3 fatty acids   A group of essential polyunsaturated fats found in green algae, cold-water fish, fish oil, flaxseed oil, and some other nut and vegetable oils. Omega 3 fatty acids have an anti-inflammatory effect on body systems.

Omega-6 fatty acids   A group of essential polyunsaturated fats found in many vegetable oils and also in meats from animals fed corn, soybeans and certain other vegetable products. Omega 6 fatty acids have an inflammatory downstream effect on body systems.

Oxidative stress   The condition in which the production of reactive oxygen species (ROS) through various metabolic pathways is at a greater rate than the body's defense system of antioxidants can handle, resulting in cellular damage at the molecular level. Oxidative stress is thought to play a part in many disease processes.

Partially hydrogenated oil   Oil that has been solidified using a catalytic chemical manufacturing process. See *trans fats*.

Peripheral neuropathy   Nerve damage caused by chronically high blood sugar. It leads to numbness, loss of sensation, and sometimes pain in the feet, legs, or hands. It is the most common complication of diabetes.

Plaque   A buildup in the arteries of cholesterol, fat, calcium, and other substances that can block blood flow and result in a heart attack or stroke.

Polycystic ovary syndrome (PCOS)   A common endocrine system disorder among women of reproductive age. Symptoms include infrequent or prolonged menstrual periods, excess hair growth, acne, and obesity. Women with PCOS tend to be insulin resistant as well.

Polydipsia   Excessive thirst.

Polyunsaturated fatty acids (PUFA)   Fats with a chemical structure that keeps them liquid in the cold; oils from corn, soybean, sunflower, safflower, cottonseed, grape seed, flaxseed, sesame seed, some nuts, and fatty fish are typically high in polyunsaturated fat.

Polyuria   Excessive urination.

Postprandial   Medical term for "after a meal."

Prediabetes   A condition in which blood-sugar levels are higher than normal but fall short of full-blown diabetes.

Protein   One of the three macronutrients found in food, used for energy and building blocks of cells. Proteins are made up of chains of amino acids, the building blocks of protein. Examples are meats, poultry, fish, shellfish, tofu and whey.

RDA (recommended daily allowance)   The average daily dietary-intake level of a nutrient that is sufficient to meet the nutrient requirements of nearly all healthy individuals (approximately 98%).

Reactive hypoglycemia   An episode of symptomatic low blood sugar which occurs about 4 hours after consuming a high-carbohydrate meal. In response to the blood-sugar spike caused by the large influx of carbohydrate, the pancreas releases an excessive surge of insulin which drives blood-glucose levels below the pre-meal baseline.

Reactive oxygen species (ROS)   Chemically reactive molecules containing oxygen, which, when produced in large amounts in the cell plasma and mitochondrial electron transport chain, can cause oxidative damage to cellular DNA and other structures and can result in cell death.

Resistance exercise   Any exercise that builds muscle strength; also called weight-bearing, weight lifting or anaerobic exercise.

Retinopathy   Damage to the retina of the eye caused by chronically high blood sugars.

ROS   See *reactive oxygen species.*

rt-CGM   Real-time continuous glucose monitor. See *CGM.*

SAD   Standard American diet, which is high in carbohydrate and lower in fat.

Satiety   A pleasurable sense of fullness.

Saturated fatty acids (SFA)   Fatty acids that are solid at room temperature; the majority of fat in butter, lard, suet, palm and coconut oil.

Serum blood sugar   Blood sugar measured from centrifuged blood taken and processed in a lab, as opposed to a whole-blood measurement done at home.

SMBG   Self-monitored blood glucose.

Substrate   In chemistry, a substance that is acted upon in a biochemical reaction, or a substance used or needed to create a new molecule.

Sucrose   Table sugar; sucrose is composed of two monosaccharides or simple sugars called glucose and fructose.

Sugar alcohols   Sweeteners, such as glycerin, mannitol, erythritol, sorbitol, and xylitol, that typically have little or no impact on blood sugar. Some are, however, anti-keto-genic in that they interfere with ketosis.

Symptomatic   Having symptoms.

T1DM (type 1 diabetes)   Type 1 diabetes mellitus, or insulin dependent diabetes mellitus (IDDM), formerly known as juvenile diabetes because it was mostly found in children. Type 1 diabetes is an autoimmune disease in which the cells that secrete insulin in the pancreas have been damaged or destroyed. The result is that the body is unable to make insulin so it must be supplied from external sources.

T2DM (type 2 diabetes) Type 2 diabetes mellitus, or non-insulin dependent diabetes mellitus (NIDDM). This condition was formerly known as adult onset diabetes because it was rarely found in children. In contrast to T1DM, type 2 manifests due to insulin resistance. The pancreas may still produce insulin, but cells have become resistant to insulin's message. In other words, the cells cannot "hear" the insulin asking to move sugar into the cells. As a result, the body cannot respond to insulin requests to move blood sugar into the cells, and the sugar in the bloodstream rises to damaging levels.

T-cell A type of white blood cell called a lymphocyte, which is part of the human immune system. There are several different kinds, each with a distinct immune system function.

Titrate To gradually increase the dose of a drug until it reaches maximum effectiveness, not necessarily the maximum dose.

Trans fats (TFA) Trans fatty acids or trans fats are found in hydrogenated or partially hydrogenated vegetable oil, typically used in fried foods, baked goods and other products. A high intake of trans fats is associated with increased risk of heart attack.

Triglycerides The major form of fat that is circulated in the bloodstream in VLDL and LDL particles and is stored as body fat. A high-carbohydrate diet increases triglycerides. Triglycerides are used as an energy source in addition to glucose, however, chronically elevated levels of triglycerides are associated with greater risks for heart disease and are a marker for insulin resistance and metabolic syndrome.

Unsaturated fat Monounsaturated fats, such as olive oil and polyunsaturated fats, found in most vegetable and fish oils. They are usually liquid at room temperature.

VLDL cholesterol Very-low-density lipoprotein. Molecules secreted by the liver that enable fats and cholesterol to move within the water-based solution of the bloodstream.

Math Symbols

<	less than
>	greater than
≠	not equal to
≤	less than or equal to
≥	greater than or equal to
±	plus or minus

Endnotes

1 Newburgh LH, Marsh PL. The use of a high fat diet in the treatment of diabetes mellitus: second paper: blood sugar. *Arch Intern Med* (chic). 1921;27(6):699–705.

2 Center for Disease Control webpage on diabetes statistics and data. Available at http://www.cdc.gov/diabetes/data/statistics/2014StatisticsReport.html

3 Cahill GF, Jr. Fuel metabolism in starvation. *Annu Rev Nutr.* 2006;26:1–22. Review.

4 Veech RL. The therapeutic implications of ketone bodies: the effects of ketone bodies in pathological conditions: ketosis, ketogenic diet, redox states, insulin resistance, and mitochondrial metabolism. *Prostaglandins Leukot Essent Fatty Acids.* 2004 Mar;70(3):309–9. Review.

5 Yamagishi, S., & Matsui, T. (2010). Advanced glycation end products, oxidative stress and diabetic nephropathy. *Oxidative Medicine and Cellular Longevity*, 3(2), 101–108. doi:10.4161/oxim.3.2.4.

6 Ahsan H. Diabetic retinopathy: Biomolecules and multiple pathophysiology. *Diabetes Metab Syndr.* 2015 January–March;9(1):51–54.

7 Sandireddy R, Yerra VG, Areti A, Komirishetty P, Kumar A. Neuroinflammation and oxidative stress in diabetic neuropathy: futuristic strategies based on these targets. *Int J Endocrinol.* 2014;2014:674987.

8 Yamagishi S. Advanced glycation end products and receptor-oxidative stress system in diabetic vascular complications. *Ther Apher Dial.* 2009 Dec;13(6):534–9.

9 Paoli A, Rubini A, Volek JS, Grimaldi KA. Beyond weight loss: a review of the therapeutic uses of very-low-carbohydrate (ketogenic) diets. *Eur J Clin Nutr.* 2013 Aug;67(8):789–96.

10 Feinman, RD, Pogozelski WK, Astrup A, Bernstein RK, Fine EJ, et al. Dietary carbohydrate restriction as the first approach in diabetes management: critical review and evidence base. *Nutrition.* 2015 Jan;31(1):1–13.

11 Center for Disease Control webpage on diabetes statistics and data. Available at http://www.cdc.gov/diabetes/data/statistics/2014StatisticsReport.html.

12 Although not discussed in this book, additional types of diabetes include gestational diabetes, a form of glucose intolerance (abnormal increase in blood glucose after a carbohydrate-containing meal or during an oral glucose-tolerance test) diagnosed during the second or third trimester of pregnancy, and type 3 diabetes, also known as Alzheimer's disease. See: de la Monte SM. Type 3 diabetes is sporadic Alzheimer's disease: mini-review. *Eur Neuropsychopharmacol.* 2014 Dec;24(12):1954-60.

13 Eades, M. A Spoonful of Sugar. Protein Power blog. Available at http://www.proteinpower.com/drmike/sugar-and-sweeteners/a-spoonful-of-sugar/

14 Symons TB, Schutzler SE, Cocke TL, Chinkes DL, Wolfe RR, Paddon-Jones D. Aging does not impair the anabolic response to a protein-rich meal. *Am J Clin Nutr.* 2007 Aug;86(2):451–6.

15 Nielsen JV, Gando C, Joensson E, Paulsson C. Low carbohydrate diet in type 1 diabetes, long-term improvement and adherence: A clinical audit. *Diabetol Metab Syndr.* 2012 May 31;4(1):23.

16 Dashti HM, Mathew TC, Khadada M, Al-Mousawi M, Talib H, Asfar SK, Behbahani AI, Al-Zaid NS. Beneficial effects of ketogenic diet in obese diabetic subjects. *Mol Cell Biochem.* 2007 Aug;302(1–2):249–56. Epub 2007 Apr 20.

17 Forsythe CE, Phinney SD, Fernandez ML, Quann EE, Wood RJ, Bibus DM, Kraemer WJ, Feinman RD, Volek JS. Comparison of low-fat and low-carbohydrate diets on circulating fatty acid composition and markers of inflammation. *Lipids.* 2008 Jan;43(1):65–77.

18 Austin GL, Thiny MT, Westman EC, Yancy WS Jr, Shaheen NJ. A very low-carbohydrate diet improves gastroesophageal reflux and its symptoms. *Dig Dis Sci.* 2006 Aug;51(8):1307–12. Epub 2006 Jul 27.

19 Struzycka I. The oral microbiome in dental caries. *Pol J Microbiol.* 2014;63(2):127–35. Review.

20 Phelps JR, Siemers SV, El-Mallakh RS. The ketogenic diet for type II bipolar disorder. *Neurocase.* 2013;19(5):423–6.

21 Kraft BD, Westman EC. Schizophrenia, gluten, and low-carbohydrate, ketogenic diets: a case report and review of the literature. *Nutr Metab (Lond).* 2009 Feb 26;6:10.

22 Giovannucci E. Metabolic syndrome, hyperinsulinemia, and colon cancer: a review. *Am J Clin Nutr.* 2007 Sep;86(3):s836–42. Review.

23 Browning JD, Baker JA, Rogers T, Davis J, Satapati S, Burgess SC. Short-term weight loss and hepatic triglyceride reduction: evidence of a metabolic advantage with dietary carbohydrate restriction. *Am J Clin Nutr.* 2011 May;93(5):1048–52.

24 Siri-Tarino PW, Sun Q, Hu FB, Krauss RM. Meta-analysis of prospective cohort studies evaluating the association of saturated fat with cardiovascular disease. *Am J Clin Nutr.* 2010 Mar;91(3):535–46.

25 Gardner CD, Kiazand A, Alhassan S, Kim S, Stafford RS, Balise RR, Kraemer HC, King AC. Comparison of the Atkins, Zone, Ornish, and LEARN diets for change in weight and related risk factors among overweight premenopausal women: the A TO Z Weight Loss Study: a randomized trial. *JAMA.* 2007 Mar 7;297(9):969–77. Erratum in: *JAMA.* 2007 Jul 11;298(2):178.

26 Sharman MJ, Kraemer WJ, Love DM, Avery NG, Gómez AL, Scheett TP, Volek JS. A ketogenic diet favorably affects serum biomarkers for cardiovascular disease in normal-weight men. *J Nutr.* 2002 Jul;132(7):1879–85.

27 Porter FD. Smith-Lemli-Opitz syndrome: pathogenesis, diagnosis and management. *Eur J Hum Genet.* 2008 May;16(5):535–41.

28 Chowdhury R, Warnakula S, Kunutsor S, Crowe F, Ward HA, et al. Association of dietary, circulating, and supplement fatty acids with coronary risk: a systematic review and meta-analysis. *Ann Intern Med.* 2014 Mar 18;160(6):398–406. doi: 10.7326/M13-1788. Review. Erratum in: *Ann Intern Med.* 2014 May 6;160(9):658.

29 Khaw KT, Wareham N, Luben R, Bingham S, Oakes S, Welch A, Day N. Glycated haemoglobin, diabetes, and mortality in men in Norfolk cohort of European prospective investigation of cancer and nutrition (EPIC-Norfolk). *BMJ.* 2001 Jan 6;322(7277):15–8.

30 Siri-Tarino PW, Sun Q, Hu FB, Krauss RM. Saturated fat, carbohydrate, and cardiovascular disease. *The American Journal of Clinical Nutrition.* 2010;91(3):502–509.

31 *Dietary Reference Intakes for Energy, Carbohydrate, Fiber, Fat, Fatty Acids, Cholesterol, Protein, and Amino Acids (Macronutrients) (2005).* The National Academies Press. Available at http://www.nap.edu/catalog/10490/dietary-reference-intakes-for-energy-carbohydrate-fiber-fat-fatty-acids-cholesterol-protein-and-amino-acids-macronutrients.

32 Kossoff EH, Freeman JM, Turner Z, Rubenstein JE. *Ketogenic diets: treatments for epilepsy and other disorders.* 5th edition. New York: Demos; 2011.

33 Saslow LR, Kim S, Daubenmier JJ, et al., A Randomized Pilot Trial of a Moderate Carbohydrate Diet Compared to a Very Low Carbohydrate Diet in Overweight or Obese Individuals with Type 2 Diabetes Mellitus or Prediabetes. Song Y, ed. *PLoS ONE.* 2014;9(4):e91027.

34 Tack C, Pohlmeier H, Behnke T, et al., Accuracy Evaluation of Five Blood Glucose Monitoring Systems Obtained from the Pharmacy: A European Multicenter Study with 453 Subjects. *Diabetes Technology & Therapeutics.* 2012;14(4):330–337. Available at http://www.ncbi.nlm.nih.gov/pmc/articles/PMC3317395/.

35 Rosedale, Ron. Cholesterol is Not the Cause of Heart Disease. Available at http://drrosedale.com/Cholesterol_is_NOT_the_cause_of_heart_disease.htm#axzz2SrJlxxHT

36 Campbell-McBride N. Cholesterol, Friend or Foe? Article available at http://www.westonaprice.org/health-topics/cholesterol-friend-or-foe/.

37 Salas-Salvadó J, Casas-Agustench P, Murphy MM, López-Uriarte P, Bulló M. The effect of nuts on inflammation. *Asia Pac J Clin Nutr.* 2008;17 Suppl 1:333–6.Review.

38 Cordain L, Miller JB, Eaton SB, Mann N, Holt SH, Speth JD. Plant-animal subsistence ratios and macronutrient energy estimations in worldwide hunter-gatherer diets. *Am J Clin Nutr.* 2000 Mar;71(3):682–92.

39 Boden et al. Effect of a low-carbohydrate diet on appetite, blood glucose levels, and insulin resistance in obese patients with type 2 diabetes. *Ann Intern Med.* 2005 Mar 15;142(6):403–11. .

40 Meijer K, de Vos P, Priebe MG. Butyrate and other short-chain fatty acids as modulators of immunity: what relevance for health? *Curr Opin Clin Nutr Metab Care.* 2010 Nov;13(6):715–21.

41 Marlett JA, Fischer MH. The active fraction of psyllium seed husk. *Proc Nutr Soc.* 2003 Feb;62(1):207–9. Review.

42 Davis E. Sugar Alcohols. Ketogenic Diet Resource. Available at http://www.ketogenic-diet-resource.com/sugar-alcohol.html.

43 CI Medical Center website. Available at http://www.cimedicalcenter.com/metabolism-p124

44 Chandalia M, Garg A, Lutjohann D, von Bergmann K, Grundy SM, Brinkley LJ. Beneficial effects of high dietary fiber intake in patients with type 2 diabetes mellitus. *N Engl J Med.* 2000 May 11;342(19):1392-8.

45 Attia, P. My Personal Nutrition Journey. Eating Academy Website. Available at http://eatingacademy.com/my-personal-nutrition-journey

46 Grundy S.M., Brewer H.B. Jr., Cleeman J.I., Smith S.C. Jr., Lenfant C., American Heart Association, National Heart Lung and Blood Institute. Definition of metabolic syndrome: Report

of the National Heart, Lung, and Blood Institute/American Heart Association conference on scientific issues related to definition. *Circulation* 2004;109:433–438.

47   Mozumdar G, Liquori G. Persistent Increase of Prevalence of Metabolic Syndrome Among U.S. Adults: NHANES III to NHANES 1999–2006. *Diabetes Care.* 2011 Jan; 34(1): 216–219.

48   Tirosh A, Shai I, Tekes-Manova D, Israeli E, Pereg D, Shochat T, Kochba I, Rudich A; Israeli Diabetes Research Group. Normal fasting plasma glucose levels and type 2 diabetes in young men. *N Engl J Med.* 2005 Oct 6;353(14):1454-62. Erratum in: *N Engl J Med.* 2006 Jun 1;354(22):2401.

49   Nichols GA, Hillier TA, Brown JB. Normal fasting plasma glucose and risk of type 2 diabetes diagnosis. *Am J Med.* 2008 Jun;121(6):519–24.

50   Bjørnholt JV, Erikssen G, Aaser E, Sandvik L, Nitter-Hauge S, Jervell J, Erikssen J, Thaulow E. Fasting blood glucose: an underestimated risk factor for cardiovascular death. Results from a 22-year follow-up of healthy nondiabetic men. *Diabetes Care.* 1999 Jan;22(1):45–9.

51   Diagnosing Diabetes and Learning About Prediabetes. American Diabetes Association website. http://www.diabetes.org/diabetes-basics/diagnosis/

52   Standards of Medical Care in Diabetes 2016. American Diabetes Association. Available at http://care.diabetesjournals.org/content/suppl/2015/12/21/39.Supplement_1.DC2/2016-Standards-of-Care.pdf

53   Handelsman et al. American Association Of Clinical Endocrinologists and American College Of Endocrinology – Clinical Practice Guidelines for Developing a Diabetes Mellitus Comprehensive Care Plan – 2015. Available at https://www.aace.com/files/dm-guidelines-ccp.pdf

54   A1C Goals, Glycemic Targets, Standards of Medical Care in Diabetes 2017. American Diabetes Association Position Statement. Available at http://care.diabetesjournals.org/content/40/Supplement_1/S48

55   Yeh HC, Brown TT, Maruthur N, Ranasinghe P, Berger Z, Suh YD, Wilson LM, Haberl EB, Brick J, Bass EB, Golden SH. Comparative effectiveness and safety of methods of insulin delivery and glucose monitoring for diabetes mellitus: a systematic review and meta-analysis. *Ann Intern Med.* 2012 Sep 4;157(5):336–47.

56   Poolsup N, Suksomboon N, Kyaw AM. Systematic review and meta-analysis of the effectiveness of continuous glucose monitoring (CGM) on glucose control in diabetes. *Diabetology & Metabolic Syndrome.* 2013;5:39.

57   Battelino T, Phillip M, Bratina N, Nimri R, Oskarsson P, Bolinder J. Effect of continuous glucose monitoring on hypoglycemia in type 1 diabetes. *Diabetes Care.* 2011 Apr;34(4):795–800. Epub 2011 Feb 19.

58   Blood Sugar Log Booklet. Wisconsin Diabetes Info. Available at http://www.ketogenic-diet-resource.com/support-files/p00246.pdf

59   American Diabetes Association. Classification and diagnosis of diabetes. Sec. 2. In Standards of Medical Care in Diabetes – 2015. *Diabetes Care* 2015;38(Suppl. 1):S8–S16.

60   American Association Of Clinical Endocrinologists and American College Of Endocrinology – Clinical Practice Guidelines For Developing A Diabetes Mellitus Comprehensive Care Plan – 2015. *Endocr Pract.* 2015;21(Suppl 1).

61 Martin-Timon I., Del Canizo-Gomez F.J. Mechanisms of hypoglycemia unawareness and implications in diabetic patients. *World J. Diabetes.* 2015;6:912–926.

62 Yun JS, Ko SH. Avoiding or coping with severe hypoglycemia in patients with type 2 diabetes. *Korean J Intern Med.* 2015 Jan;30(1):6–16.

63 Daly ME, Vale C, Walker M, Littlefield A, Alberti KG, Mathers JC. Acute effects on insulin sensitivity and diurnal metabolic profiles of a high-sucrose compared with a high-starch diet. *Am J Clin Nutr.* 1998 Jun;67(6):1186–96.

64 Borg R, Kuenen JC, Carstensen B, et al. HbA1c and mean blood glucose show stronger associations with cardiovascular disease risk factors than do postprandial glycaemia or glucose variability in persons with diabetes: the A1C-Derived Average Glucose (ADAG) study. *Diabetologia.* 2011;54(1):69–72.

65 Goldin A, Beckman JA, Schmidt AM, Creager MA. Advanced glycation end products: sparking the development of diabetic vascular injury. *Circulation.* 2006 Aug 8;114(6):597–605. Review.

66 Forbes JM, Cooper ME. Glycation in diabetic nephropathy. *Amino Acids.* 2012 Apr;42(4):1185–92. Epub 2010 Oct 21. Review. .

67 Sugimoto K, Yasujima M, Yagihashi S. Role of advanced glycation end products in diabetic neuropathy. *Curr Pharm Des.* 2008;14(10):953–61. Review.

68 Stitt AW. The role of advanced glycation in the pathogenesis of diabetic retinopathy. *Exp Mol Pathol.* 2003 Aug;75(1):95–108. Review.

69 The effect of intensive treatment of diabetes on the development and progression of long-term complications in insulin-dependent diabetes mellitus. The Diabetes Control and Complications Trial Research Group. *N Engl J Med.* 1993 Sep 30;329(14):977–86.

70 Koga M, Kasayama S. Clinical impact of glycated albumin as another glycemic control marker. *Endocr J.* 2010;57(9):751–62. Epub 2010 Aug 17. Review.

71 390 Drugs that Affect Blood Sugar. Diabetes in Control website. Diabetes in Control website. Available at http://www.diabetesincontrol.com/tools/tools-for-your-practice/9625-drugs-that-can-affect-blood-glucose-levels.

72 CI Medical Center Metabolism and BMR Calculator. Available at http://www.cimedicalcenter.com/metabolism-calculating-your-bmr-bmi-p124.

73 Sapir DG, Owen OE. Renal conservation of ketone bodies during starvation. *Metabolism.* 1975 Jan;24(1):23–33.

74 Schwartz RM, Boyes S, Aynsley-Green A. Metabolic effects of three ketogenic diets in the treatment of severe epilepsy. *Dev Med Child Neurol.* 1989 Apr;31(2):152–60.

75 Reichard GA Jr, Owen OE, Haff AC, Paul P, Bortz WM. Ketone-body production and oxidation in fasting obese humans. *J Clin Invest.* 1974 Feb;53(2):508–15.

76 Runyan, K. Ketogenic Diabetic Athlete Blog. Available at https://ketogenicdiabeticathlete.wordpress.com.

77 Triplitt C. Drug interactions of medications commonly used in diabetes. Diabetes Spectr2006;19:202–11.

78 Kasim SE. Dietary marine fish oils and insulin action in type 2 diabetes. *Ann NY Acad Sci.* 1993 Jun 14;683:250–7. Review.

79 Borkman M, Chisholm DJ, Furler SM, Storlien LH, Kraegen EW, Simons LA, Chesterman CN. Effects of fish oil supplementation on glucose and lipid metabolism in NIDDM. *Diabetes.* 1989 Oct;38(10):1314–9.

80 Misbin RI. The phantom of lactic acidosis due to metformin in patients with diabetes. *Diabetes Care.* 2004 Jul;27(7):1791–3. Review.

81 Ekström N, Schiöler L, Svensson A-M, et al. Effectiveness and safety of metformin in 51, 675 patients with type 2 diabetes and different levels of renal function: a cohort study from the Swedish National Diabetes Register. *BMJ Open.* 2012;2(4):e001076.

82 Takahashi, Akira et al. Sulfonylurea and glinide reduce insulin content, functional expression of KATP channels, and accelerate apoptotic β-cell death in the chronic phase. *Diabetes Research and Clinical Practice*, Volume 77, Issue 3, 343–350.

83 Pantalone KM, Kattan MW, Yu C, Wells BJ, Arrigain S, Jain A, Atreja A, Zimmerman RS. Increase in overall mortality risk in patients with type 2 diabetes receiving glipizide, glyburide or glimepiride monotherapy versus metformin: a retrospective analysis. *Diabetes Obes Metab.* 2012 Sep;14(9):803–9.

84 Home PD, Pocock SJ, Beck-Nielsen H, Curtis PS, Gomis R, Hanefeld M, Jones NP, Komajda M, McMurray JJ; RECORD Study Team. Rosiglitazone evaluated for cardiovascular outcomes in oral agent combination therapy for type 2 diabetes (RECORD): a multicentre, randomised, open-label trial. *Lancet.* 2009 Jun 20;373(9681):2125–35.

85 FDA Drug Safety Communication: Update to ongoing safety review of Actos (pioglitazone) and increased risk of bladder cancer. Available at http://www.fda.gov/drugs/drugsafety/ucm259150.htm#ref.

86 Nissen SE, Wolski K. Effect of rosiglitazone on the risk of myocardial infarction and death from cardiovascular causes. *N Engl J Med.* 2007 Jun 14;356(24):2457–71. Erratum in: *N Engl J Med.* 2007 Jul 5;357(1):100.

87 Regulation of food preference using GLP-1 agonists. Patent Application. Available at https://www.google.com/patents/EP2298337A2?cl=en.

88 Karagiannis T, Boura P, Tsapas A. Safety of dipeptidyl peptidase 4 inhibitors: a perspective review. *Ther Adv Drug Saf.* 2014 Jun;5(3):138–46.

89 Lee NJ, Norris SL, Thakurta S. Efficacy and Harms of the Hypoglycemic Agent Pramlintide in Diabetes Mellitus. *Annals of Family Medicine.* 2010;8(6):542–549.

90 Rosenstock J, Ferrannini E. Euglycemic Diabetic Ketoacidosis: A Predictable, Detectable, and Preventable Safety Concern With SGLT2 Inhibitors. *Diabetes Care.* 2015 Sep;38(9):1638–42.

91 Dehn C. SGLT inhibition in patients with type 1 diabetes. *Lancet* June 2014. Available at http://www.the*Lancet*.com/pdfs/journals/landia/PIIS2213-8587(14)70112-3.pdf.

92 Zintzaras E, Miligkos M, Ziakas P, Balk EM, Mademtzoglou D, Doxani C, et al. Assessment of the relative effectiveness and tolerability of treatments of type 2 diabetes mellitus: a network meta-analysis. *Clin Ther.* 2014 Oct 1;36(10):1443–53.e9.

93 Comparison of Insulin Preparations. Camden Health website. Available at https://www. camdenhealth.org/wp-content/uploads/2011/03/Insulin_Preparation-3-14-11.pdf

94 Stewart WJ, McSweeney SM, Kellett MA, Faxon DP, Ryan TJ. Increased risk of severe protamine reactions in NPH insulin-dependent diabetics undergoing cardiac catheterization. *Circulation*. 1984 Nov;70(5):788–92.

95 De Leeuw I, Vague P, Selam JL, Skeie S, Lang H, Draeger E, Elte JW. Insulin detemir used in basal-bolus therapy in people with type 1 diabetes is associated with a lower risk of nocturnal hypoglycaemia and less weight gain over 12 months in comparison to NPH insulin. *Diabetes Obes Metab*. 2005 Jan;7(1):73–82.

96 Søeborg T, Rasmussen CH, Mosekilde E, Colding-Jørgensen M. Bioavailability and variability of biphasic insulin mixtures. *Eur J Pharm Sci*. 2012 Jul 16;46(4):198–208. Epub 2011 Jun 16. Review.

97 Marran KJ, Davey B, Lang A, Segal DG. Exponential increase in postprandial blood-glucose exposure with increasing carbohydrate loads using a linear carbohydrate-to-insulin ratio. *S Afr Med J*. 2013 Apr 10;103(7):461-3

98 Bell, Kirstine J et al. Efficacy of carbohydrate counting in type 1 diabetes: a systematic review and meta-analysis. The *Lancet Diabetes & Endocrinology*, Volume 2, Issue 2, 133–140.

99 Bergenstal RM, Johnson M, Powers MA, Wynne A, Vlajnic A, Hollander P, Rendell M. Adjust to target in type 2 diabetes: comparison of a simple algorithm with carbohydrate counting for adjustment of mealtime insulin glulisine. *Diabetes Care*. 2008 Jul;31(7):1305–10.

100 Laurenzi A, Bolla AM, Panigoni G, et al. Effects of Carbohydrate Counting on Glucose Control and Quality of Life Over 24 Weeks in Adult Patients With Type 1 Diabetes on Continuous Subcutaneous Insulin Infusion: A randomized, prospective clinical trial (GIOCAR). *Diabetes Care*. 2011;34(4):823–827. doi:10.2337/dc10-1490.

101 Johnson SR, Cooper MN, Jones TW, Davis EA. Long-term outcome of insulin pump therapy in children with type 1 diabetes assessed in a large population-based case-control study. *Diabetologia*. 2013 Nov;56(11):2392–400. Epub 2013 Aug 21.

102 Plank J, Bodenlenz M, Sinner F, Magnes C, Görzer E, Regittnig W et al. A double-blind, randomized, dose-response study investigating the pharmacodynamic and pharmacokinetic properties of the long-acting insulin analog detemir. *Diabetes Care*. 2005 May;28(5):1107–12.

103 Layman DK. Dietary Guidelines should reflect new understandings about adult protein needs. *Nutrition & Metabolism*. 2009;6:12.

104 Volek JS, Phinney SD, Forsythe CE, Quann EE, Wood RJ, Puglisi MJ, Kraemer WJ, Bibus DM, Fernandez ML, Feinman RD. Carbohydrate restriction has a more favorable impact on the metabolic syndrome than a low fat diet. *Lipids*. 2009 Apr;44(4):297–309.

105 Borghouts LB, Keizer HA. Exercise and insulin sensitivity: a review. *Int J Sports Med*. 2000 Jan;21(1):1–12. Review.

106 King DS, Baldus PJ, Sharp RL, Kesl LD, Feltmeyer TL, Riddle MS. Time course for exercise-induced alterations in insulin action and glucose tolerance in middle-aged people. *J Appl Physiol* (1985). 1995 Jan;78(1):17–22.

107 Lumb A. Diabetes and exercise. *Clinical Medicine* 2014; 14 (6): 63–6.

108 Hainer V, Stunkard A, Kunesová M, Parízková J, Stich V, Allison DB. A twin study of weight loss and metabolic efficiency. *Int J Obes Relat Metab Disord*. 2001 Apr;25(4):533–7.

109 van der Heijden GJ, Sauer PJ, Sunehag AL. Twelve weeks of moderate aerobic exercise without dietary intervention or weight loss does not affect 24-h energy expenditure in lean and obese adolescents. *Am J Clin Nutr*. 2010 Mar;91(3):589–96.

110 Cuff DJ, Meneilly GS, Martin A, Ignaszewski A, Tildesley HD, Frohlich JJ. Effective exercise modality to reduce insulin resistance in women with type 2 diabetes. *Diabetes Care*. 2003 Nov;26(11):2977–82.

111 Borghouts LB, Keizer HA. Exercise and insulin sensitivity: a review. *Int J Sports Med*. 2000 Jan;21(1):1–12. Review.

112 Dhaliwal SS, Welborn TA, Howat PA. Recreational Physical Activity as an Independent Predictor of Multivariable Cardiovascular Disease Risk. Moro C, ed. PLoS ONE. 2013;8(12):e83435.

113 Volek JS, Freidenreich DJ, Saenz C, Kunces LJ, Creighton BC, Bartley JM, et al. Metabolic characteristics of keto-adapted ultra-endurance runners. *Metabolism*. 2016 Mar;65(3):100–10.

114 Phinney SD, Bistrian BR, Wolfe RR, Blackburn GL. The human metabolic response to chronic ketosis without caloric restriction: physical and biochemical adaptation. *Metabolism*. 1983 Aug;32(8):757–68.

115 Timothy Allen Olson website. Available at http://www.timothyallenolson.com/tag/western-states

116 Zach Bittern website. Available at http://zachbitterrunning.blogspot.com/p/results.html

117 Gibala MJ, Gillen JB, Percival ME. Physiological and Health-Related Adaptations to Low-Volume Interval Training: Influences of Nutrition and Sex. *Sports Medicine* (Auckland, N.z). 2014;44(Suppl 2):127–137.

118 Kuehnbaum NL, Gillen JB, Gibala MJ, Britz-McKibbin P. Personalized Metabolomics for Predicting Glucose Tolerance Changes in Sedentary Women After High-Intensity Interval Training. *Scientific Report*s. 2014;4:6166.

119 Motahari-Tabari N, Ahmad Shirvani M, Shirzad-E-Ahoodashty M, Yousefi-Abdolmaleki E, Teimourzadeh M. The effect of 8 weeks aerobic exercise on insulin resistance in type 2 diabetes: a randomized clinical trial. *Glob J Health Sci*. 2014 Aug 14;7(1):115–21.

120 Cuff DJ, Meneilly GS, Martin A, Ignaszewski A, Tildesley HD, Frohlich JJ. Effective exercise modality to reduce insulin resistance in women with type 2 diabetes. *Diabetes Care*. 2003 Nov;26(11):2977–82.

121 Knowler WC, Bennett PH, Hamman RF, Miller M. Diabetes incidence and prevalence in Pima Indians: a 19-fold greater incidence than in Rochester, Minnesota. *Am J Epidemiol*. 1978 Dec;108(6):497–505.

122 The United States Farm Subsidy Information. Environmental Working Group website. Available at http://farm.ewg.org/region.php?fips=00000

123 2015–2020 Dietary Guidelines for Americans. Health.gov website. Available at https://health.gov/dietaryguidelines/2015/default.asp

124 Sulfonylureas, meglitinides, thiazolidinediones, and insulin can result in weight gain when consuming a typical ADA recommended carbohydrate diet. Sulfonylureas, meglitinides, amylin

mimetics, and insulin can cause hypoglycemia, whereas metformin, thiazolidinediones, GLP-1 agonists, DPP-4 inhibitors, and SGLT2 inhibitors do not by themselves. SGLT2 inhibitors increase the risk of diabetic ketoacidosis.

125 Cahill GF Jr, Herrera MG, Morgan AP, Soeldner JS, Steinke J, Levy PL, Reichard GA Jr, Kipnis DM. Hormone-fuel interrelationships during fasting. *J Clin Invest.* 1966 Nov;45(11):1751–69.

126 Cahill GF, Aoki TT, Ruderman NB. Ketosis. Transactions of the American Clinical and Climatological Association. 1973;84:184–202.

127 McCue, Marshall D. (Ed.) Comparative Physiology of Fasting, Starvation, and Food Limitation. Chapter 2: Lignot J, LeMaho Y. *A History of Modern Research in Fasting, Starvation and Ination.* Springer, 2012, XIV, 430 pages.

128 Stewart WK, Fleming LW. Features of a successful therapeutic fast of 382 days' duration. *Postgraduate Medical Journal.* 1973;49(569):203–209.

Acknowledgments

Many thanks to Miriam Kalamian, for both her assistance and her expertise in implementing ketogenic diets and for being a good friend and mentor to me. Thanks also to Amy Berger for her friendship and for her time, knowledge, and suggestions for improving this book. Thanks also go to editor Annie Jo Smith for her excellent work and suggestions, and to Dr. Keith Runyan, whose contributions have made this a truly unique and useful book.

I would also like to thank the researchers and authors who are working to bring the truth about the efficacy of treating diabetes with a low-carb ketogenic diet to the public despite the resistance of national diabetes organizations and pharmaceutical companies. My thanks go to Richard D. Feinman, PhD; Wendy K. Pogozelski, PhD; Arne Astrup, MD; Richard K. Bernstein, MD; Eugene J. Fine, MS, MD; Eric C. Westman, MD, MHS; Anthony Accurso, MD; Lynda Frassetto, MD; Barbara A. Gower, PhD; Samy I. McFarlane, MD; Jörgen Vesti Nielsen, MD; Thure Krarup, MD; Laura Saslow, PhD; Karl S. Roth, MD; Mary C. Vernon, MD; Jeff S. Volek, RD, PhD; Gilbert B. Wilshire, MD; Annika Dahlqvist, MD; Ralf Sundberg, MD, PhD; Ann Childers, MD; Katharine Morrison, MRCGP; Anssi H. Manninen, MHS; Hussain M. Dashti, MD, PhD, FACS, FICS; Richard J. Wood, PhD; Jay Wortman, MD; Keith Runyan, MD; Stephen D. Phinney, MD, PhD; Nicolai Worm, PhD; Gary Taubes; Peter Attia, MD; Jeff Gerber, MD; Andreas Eenfeldt, MD; David Mendosa; Ron Rosedale, MD; Jenny Ruhl; and Jason Fung, MD.

Finally, thank you to everyone spends time reading our websites and books. We appreciate your attention, and hope the information helps you to achieve excellent health.

About the Authors

Ellen Davis has a Master's degree in Applied Clinical Nutrition from New York Chiropractic College. She created Ketogenic-Diet-Resource.com, a website showcasing the research on the positive health effects of ketogenic diets. Ellen has written articles for Well Being Journal, Terry's Naturally magazine and Healthy Living magazine, and authored several other books, including her book *The Ketogenic Diet for Type 1 Diabetes,* also coauthored with Keith Runyan, MD. In addition, her book *Fight Cancer with a Ketogenic Diet* is helping cancer patients utilize a ketogenic diet as therapy in over 70 countries.

Keith Runyan is medical doctor who has practiced clinical medicine in the areas of emergency medicine, internal medicine, nephrology, and obesity medicine. In 1998, he was diagnosed with type 1 diabetes and subsequently followed the conventional advice to treat his condition for the next 14 years. Although his glycemic control was at "recommended levels" of HbA1c of 6.5-7%, he was disturbed by frequent hypoglycemic episodes. After starting regular exercise to train for triathlons in 2007, his glycemic control actually worsened from taking sports gels to prevent hypoglycemia. When he contemplated doing an ironman distance triathlon in 2011, he sought a better method to control his diabetes. He came across the ketogenic diet in 2012 and experienced a rapid and remarkable improvement not only in glycemic control, but also in preventing hypoglycemia and its symptoms. He completed the ironman distance triathlon in 2012 without sugar, food, or hypoglycemia while in nutritional ketosis. He is now an advocate for the use of the ketogenic diet for management of diabetes and has authored books explaining its use and benefits for diabetes. He documents his results on his blog at ketogenicdiabeticathlete.wordpress.com.

Visit

www.ketogenic-diet-resource.com

for more information on ketogenic diet
research and applications, and to purchase
our other books:

*Fight Cancer with a
Ketogenic Diet*

*The Ketogenic Diet for
Type 1 Diabetes*

and Dr. Runyan's blog:

ketogenicdiabeticathlete.wordpress.com

for more information on managing diabetes.

56104040R00139

Made in the USA
Columbia, SC
20 April 2019